T0249001

Encyclopedia of Drug Discovery and Development: Today and Tomorrow

Volume I

Encyclopedia of Drug Discovery and Development: Today and Tomorrow

Volume I

Edited by **Ned Burnett**

FOSTER
A C A D E M I C S

New Jersey

Published by Foster Academics,
61 Van Reypen Street,
Jersey City, NJ 07306, USA
www.fosteracademics.com

Encyclopedia of Drug Discovery and Development: Today and Tomorrow
Volume I
Edited by Ned Burnett

International Standard Book Number: 978-1-63242-136-4 (Hardback)

This book contains information obtained from authentic and highly regarded sources. Copyright for all individual chapters remain with the respective authors as indicated. A wide variety of references are listed. Permission and sources are indicated; for detailed attributions, please refer to the permissions page. Reasonable efforts have been made to publish reliable data and information, but the authors, editors and publisher cannot assume any responsibility for the validity of all materials or the consequences of their use.

The publisher's policy is to use permanent paper from mills that operate a sustainable forestry policy. Furthermore, the publisher ensures that the text paper and cover boards used have met acceptable environmental accreditation standards.

Trademark Notice: Registered trademark of products or corporate names are used only for explanation and identification without intent to infringe.

Printed in the United States of America.

Contents

Preface

Drug discovery and development process focuses on details regarding medications that are safe and efficient in improving the length and quality of life and relaxing pain and suffering. However, the process is very intricate, time taking, resource intensive, requiring multidisciplinary expertise and novel approaches. There is a need to identify and produce more effective and appropriate ways to bring safe and effective products to the market. Translational research is a rapidly growing discipline of biomedicine. It is a bidirectional bench-to-bedside approach, in an effort to improve the process efficacy and the need for further innovations. The book describes the contemporary and evolving state of drug discovery and development, and the existing and emerging models for evaluating efficacy and safety in drug discovery.

After months of intensive research and writing, this book is the end result of all who devoted their time and efforts in the initiation and progress of this book. It will surely be a source of reference in enhancing the required knowledge of the new developments in the area. During the course of developing this book, certain measures such as accuracy, authenticity and research focused analytical studies were given preference in order to produce a comprehensive book in the area of study.

This book would not have been possible without the efforts of the authors and the publisher. I extend my sincere thanks to them. Secondly, I express my gratitude to my family and well-wishers. And most importantly, I thank my students for constantly expressing their willingness and curiosity in enhancing their knowledge in the field, which encourages me to take up further research projects for the advancement of the area.

Editor

Introductory Chapter

Overview of Current Drug Discovery and Development with an Eye Towards the Future

Izet M. Kapetanovic

Division of Cancer Prevention, National Cancer Institute, Bethesda, MD
USA

1. Introduction

Drug discovery and development process aims to make available new pharmacological interventions to prevent, treat, mitigate, or cure disease in a safe and effective manner. It is a slow, complex, multi disciplinary and costly process. Drug development starts with a target identification and validation, followed by drug candidates (hits) discovery, and lead drug (compound with favorable pharmaceutical, safety, efficacy, and pharmacokinetic profile) selection and optimization. Preclinical (non clinical) efficacy, pharmacology, toxicology, and mechanistic studies may include *in silico* (computational) methods, use of *in vitro* animal or human tissues (including cells and subcellular fractions), and *in vivo* animals. The studies rely on models that are thought to be predictive of the subsequent preclinical or clinical effects. Guidances (government-regulated standards of normal expectations) for different steps are readily available from the regulatory agencies (http://www.fda.gov/drugs/guidancecomplianceregulatoryinformation/guidances/default.htm). The required toxic ology studies must be performed according to the Good Laboratory Practice (GLP) guidelines. Medicinal chemistry and pharmaceutics also play a crucial role from the beginning of the drug discovery and development process, involving chemical synthesis (including compliance with current Good Manufacturing Practice, cGMP), characterization, purification, chemical alteration, stability determination, and formulation of the drug candidate. The first-in-human (FIH) doses are based on the No-Observed-Adverse-Event-Level (NOAEL) values obtained in the relevant and more sensitive toxicology specie (rodent and non-rodent, commonly rat and dog), interspecies dose extrapolation, and a selection of an appropriate safety factor. Subsequent to preclinical evaluation, an Investigational New Drug (IND) application is submitted to the regulatory agency (e.g. United States Food and Drug Administration, FDA or European Medicine Agency, EMEA) summarizing all preclinical data (chemical, pharmaceutical, efficacy, toxicology and other) along with a rationale for the proposed clinical study and a clinical study protocol. Clinical drug development can commence after review of the IND by the regulatory agency and a clinical study approval by a local Institutional Review Board (IRB, a committee of scientists and non-scientists overseeing the clinical research). Phase 1 studies commonly use human volunteers to determine human safety and pharmacokinetics. Frequently, these studies also include biomarkers of efficacy as secondary endpoints. Drugs with acceptable safety profiles then enter Phase 2 for efficacy evaluations. These include the proof-of-principle studies to demonstrate effects on disease-relevant biomarkers and the proof-of-concept studies to demonstrate direct effects on the target disease in a small patient sampling. Controlled trials are commonly designed to compare effects of the new drug to a placebo or to a standard of care treatment (for ethical reasons). Drugs showing promising efficacy continue to Phase 3, much larger trials examining efficacy as well as safety. Drugs emerging from these trials with appropriate evidence of safety and efficacy are submitted for marketing approval via a New Drug Application (NDA). Following a review and approval by the regulatory agency, the drug can then be marketed and enters Phase 4 or post-marketing monitoring.

Recent estimates suggest that it takes up to 13.5 years and 1.8 billion U.S. dollars to bring a new drug to the market [17]. There are rising concerns over the diminished productivity (number of new medical entities approved) in face of the escalating cost (R&D spending). In view of this, there is a growing effort and urgency to find new approaches aiming to decrease attrition and increase success in drug development [8, 10, 11, 17]. This is at times when number of drug blockbusters is coming off patent, large personnel layoffs and pharmaceutical consolidation (buying and merging in an effort to shore up pharmaceutical company pipelines). There are strong beliefs that pharmaceutical industry needs to find means of improving efficiency and effectiveness in order to sustain itself. Two independent studies, one by the FDA and the other by the European Federation of Pharmaceutical Industries and Associations (EFPIA), examined the causes behind the decreasing productivity. Based on these studies, improvements in predictivity of safety and efficacy were deemed to have the greatest potential for reversing the trend of diminished productivity and success [10]. This led to formation of public-private initiatives aiming to accelerate the development of better and safer medicines, the Innovative Medicines Initiative, IMI (http://imi.europa.eu) and the Critical Path Institute, C-PATH (http://www.c-path.org/). In 2004, FDA launched the Critical Path Initiative (CPI) as described in its white paper *Innovation/Stagnation: Challenge and Opportunity on the Critical Path to New Medical Products* (http://www.fda.gov/ScienceResearch/SpecialTopics/Critical PathInitiative/CriticalPathOpportunitiesReports/ucm077262.htm):

"Sounding the alarm on the increasing difficulty and unpredictability of medical product development, the report concluded that collective action was needed to modernize scientific and technical tools as well as harness information technology to evaluate and predict the safety, effectiveness, and manufacturability of medical products. The report called for a national effort to identify specific activities all along the critical path of medical product development and use, which, if undertaken, would help transform the critical path sciences."

This was echoed in subsequent C-PATH reports (http://www.fda.gov/downloads/ScienceResearch/SpecialTopics/CriticalPathInitiative/UCM186110.pdf;http://www.fda.gov/ScienceResearch/SpecialTopics/CriticalPathInitiative/ucm076689.htm). Dr. Raymond Woosley, the president and CEO of the C-PATH is quoted on the C-PATH's website that it presently takes 15 years for drug development and 95% of drug candidate fail along the way. The very ambitious goal cited by the Institute is to shorten the time to 3 years and improve the success to 95%.

Major reasons cited for drug attrition are lack of efficacy, presence of toxicity, and commercial concerns [12]. It was reported that only 5% of the compounds entering the first-in-human studies in oncology achieve successful registration [12]. Majority of failures occurred in Phase 3 and were attributed to the lack of efficacy proof of concept, lack of objective and robust biomarkers, inadequate predictivity and poor translation of scientific discoveries and preclinical information to clinical settings. Innovation was commonly viewed as one of the most needed approaches to reversing the situation [8, 11, 17, 24]. A recent Science editorial by the current FDA commissioner [6] echoed these viewpoints. Commonly cited areas for potential and fruitful innovations include the development process itself, identification, validation and qualification of relevant biomarkers, predictive modeling, clinical trial subject selection, clinical trial design, and collaborative efforts involving pharmaceutical companies, academia, government, and public.

"Fail fast, fail cheap" is a common mantra in the pharmaceutical industry. This is intended to minimize losses of time, resources, and expenses. There are number of go/no-go decision gates along the common drug development path. Earlier an appropriate no-go decision is made, lesser the possibility for waste. Drug developers strive to identify the most effective and efficient means of bringing safe and effective products to the market. Success along the development path hinges on using appropriate and robust models and biomarkers, which are relevant and predictive of a disease process of interest. One frequently proposed solution is to move the clinical proof-of-concept phase to an earlier point on the drug development timeline and in a bidirectional manner with the preclinical development [17]. It's expected that this would result in a lesser number of drug candidates entering later clinical testing phases but with increasing probability of their success.

In an effort to decrease the development time and improve drug development efficiency, the regulatory agencies have recently introduced the Exploratory Phase (also known as Phase 0) option(http://www.fda.gov/downloads/Drugs/GuidanceComplianceRegulatoryInformati on/Guidances/ucm078933.pdf). The regu latory requirements for Exploratory Phase are lesser than those for Phase 1 but the doses and scope of the former are also more limited. The Exploratory Phase has no therapeutic or diagnostic intent. Its purpose is to obtain pharmacokinetic and/or pharmacodynamic data and thereby provide an opportunity to obtain the necessary information for an early decision whether to continue the development or to select the optimum candidate or formulation for development [22].

One of the major initiatives in an effort to improve the efficiency and success in drug development deals with identification and validation of robust and predictive biomarkers. Biomarkers play a pivotal role throughout the drug discovery and development process, from the beginning through post-marketing. Biomarker Consortium, composed of the National Institutes of Health, the FDA, the Center for Medicare and Medicaid Services, Pharmaceutical Research and Manufacturers of America (PhRMA), Biotechnology Industry Association (BIO), pharmaceutical companies, academia, and patient groups, was formed in the United States to accelerate development in this area. Present and future perspectives by FDA on molecular biomarkers have been summarized in a recent publication [7]. The Predictive Safety Testing Consortium, PSTC (http://www.c-path.org/pstc.cfm) represents an example of one successful collaborative effort stemming from some of these initiatives. In collaboration with the regulatory agencies (FDA and EMEA), the PSTC worked on defining methodologies and validations for new safety biomarkers and presented an initial path and outline for regulatory qualification of biomarkers [5, 21]. In addition through the efforts of the Nephrotoxicity Working Group, seven renal biomarkers have been qualified for limited use in nonclinical and clinical drug development as a measure of drug safety. These efforts were highlighted in a special issue of Nature Biotechnology (http://www.natur e.com/nbt/journal/v28/n5/index.html).

Advances in hardware and software computational power and sophistication are fueling the rapidly growing reliance on computers and computational modeling in an attempt to improve the efficiency and effectiveness in the drug discovery and development process [9]. It's not uncommon to hear statements at drug development conferences that computational modeling will play the major role in drug design and development in not too distant future, similar to its role presently in the automotive and airplane industries. Computational modeling addresses the key critical element in all aspects of the drug discovery and development process, the prediction [13]. This *in silico* approach is thought to obviate some disadvantages of the more traditional approaches (need for large amounts of test agent for *in vivo* testing, poor predictability of *in vivo* animal and *in vitro* models for human toxicity and efficacy, lack of reliable high-throughput *in vitro* assays and a lack of animal models for some common adverse events seen in humans, e.g. headache, nausea, dizziness) [16]. There are also increasing legal requirements, especially in Europe, for use of alternative, non-animal models in the regulatory safety assessment of chemicals and urging development, independent assessment and application of computational methods. [15]. As stated in the *Science* editorial: "The FDA is also working to eventually replace animal testing with a combination of *in silico* and *in vitro* approaches" [6]. In 2007, the National Academy of Sciences also proposed a shift away from the current animal toxicology testing to use of emerging technologies i.e., *in vitro* assays using human cells, non-mammalian model organisms, high throughput testing, imaging technologies, omics technologies, systems biology, and computational modeling. Some of the advantages and disadvantages of these approaches were recently discussed by van Vliet [23]. In order to address the great complexity of the biological systems, extensive computational power is required and there are several major virtual screening efforts utilizing grid or distributed computing (e.g. http://www.worldcommunitygrid.org/research/hdc/overview.do). *PriceWaterhouse Coopers Pharma 2005: An Industrial Revolution in R&D* report emphasized the growth and value of *in silico* approaches and projected that *in silico* methods will become dominant from drug discovery through marketing (http://www.pwc.com/en_GX/gx/pharma-lifesciences/pdf/industrial_revolution.pdf). Furthermore, the report suggested that we are in a transitional period where the roles of primary (laboratory and clinical studies) and secondary (computational) science are in process of reversal. In a more recent report, *PriceWaterhouseCoopers Pharma 2020: Virtual R&D*, it was stated that pharmaceutical innovation and productivity could be improved significantly via enhanced and more complete molecular understanding of the human body and a more complete knowledge of human disease pathophysiology, thereby enabling development of more predictive computational models (http://www.pwc.be/en/pharma/pdf/Pharma-2020-virtual-rd-PwC-09.pdf). This was envisioned as a path towards predictive biosimulation in form of a "virtual man" and a "virtual patient" in some not too distant future with some of the effort along these lines already in progress.

The rapid growth in scientific knowledge and computational capabilities is also providing means for integrating and analyzing disparate chemical, biochemical, physiological, pathological, and clinical data in a parallel as opposed to a sequential fashion. Systems biology applies principles and mathematical tools of electrical engineering and networks to dynamic modeling and simulation of complex biological systems in a holistic manner. This is facilitating a change in drug discovery and development paradigm away from the reductionist approach. It's becoming more recognized that a commonly utilized reductionist approach may not be well suited for complex human disease processes and that the old magic bullet paradigm needs to be replaced by a magic shotgun for many of the diseases

[19]. Human physiology and pathology are very complex involving multi-factorial and heterogenous processes with dynamic, redundant and interactive networks and signaling pathways [1-4, 14, 18, 20]. In fact, the term "Network Medicine" and what it entails is growing in recognition [2]. Furthermore, one size doesn't fit all and the targets may also change as the disease progresses. In many cases, it's more relevant to understand the system and how to apply and interpret its perturbations in order to achieve desired efficacy and safety as opposed to concentrating on a single target. In fact, a partial modification of several targets may be more effective and safer than a complete modification of a single target.

Based on the above overview, it is clear that changes and innovations in drug discovery and development are needed and that there are ongoing efforts in this area on several fronts. Ultimately, the success hinges on improving the predictivity of efficacy and toxicity, which in turn depends on innovations and having reliable and robust biomarkers and using appropriate tools and methodologies.

2. References

[1] Azmi AS, Wang Z, Philip PA, Mohammad RM, Sarkar FH (2010) Proof of Concept: Network and Systems Biology Approaches Aid in the Discovery of Potent Anticancer Drug Combinations. Molecular Cancer Therapeutics 9: 3137-3144

[2] Barabási AL, Gulbahce N, Loscalzo J (2011) Network medicine: A network-based approach to human disease. Nature Reviews Genetics 12: 56-68

[3] Boran ADW, Iyengar R (2010) Systems pharmacology. Mount Sinai Journal of Medicine 77: 333-344

[4] Csermely P, Agoston V, Pongor S (2005) The efficiency of multi-target drugs: the network approach might help drug design. Trends Pharmacol Sci 26: 178-82

[5] Dieterle F, Sistare F, Goodsaid F, Papaluca M, Ozer JS, Webb CP, Baer W, Senagore A, Schipper MJ, Vonderscher J, Sultana S, Gerhold DL, Phillips JA, Maurer G, Carl K, Laurie D, Harpur E, Sonee M, Ennulat D, Holder D, Andrews-Cleavenger D, Gu YZ, Thompson KL, Goering PL, Vidal JM, Abadie E, Maciulaitis R, Jacobson-Kram D, Defelice AF, Hausner EA, Blank M, Thompson A, Harlow P, Throckmorton D, Xiao S, Xu N, Taylor W, Vamvakas S, Flamion B, Lima BS, Kasper P, Pasanen M, Prasad K, Troth S, Bounous D, Robinson-Gravatt D, Betton G, Davis MA, Akunda J, McDuffie JE, Suter L, Obert L, Guffroy M, Pinches M, Jayadev S, Blomme EA, Beushausen SA, Barlow VG, Collins N, Waring J, Honor D, Snook S, Lee J, Rossi P, Walker E, Mattes W (2010) Renal biomarker qualification submission: a dialog between the FDA-EMEA and Predictive Safety Testing Consortium. Nat Biotechnol 28: 455-62

[6] Hamburg MA (2011) Advancing regulatory science. Science 331: 987

[7] Hong H, Goodsaid F, Shi L, Tong W (2010) Molecular biomarkers: a US FDA effort. Biomark Med 4: 215-25

[8] Kaitin KI (2008) Obstacles and Opportunities in New Drug Development. Clin Pharmacol Ther 83: 210-212

[9] Kapetanovic IM (2008) Computer-aided drug discovery and development (CADDD): in silico-chemico-biological approach. Chem Biol Interact 171: 165-76

[10] Koening J (2011) Does process excellence handcuff drug development? Drug Discov Today 16: 377-381

[11] Kola I (2008) The State of Innovation in Drug Development. Clin Pharmacol Ther 83: 227-230

[12] Kola I, Landis J (2004) Can the pharmaceutical industry reduce attrition rates? Nat Rev Drug Discov 3: 711-5

[13] Kumar N, Hendriks BS, Janes KA, de Graaf D, Lauffenburger DA (2006) Applying computational modeling to drug discovery and development. Drug Discovery Today 11: 806-811

[14] Lowe JA, Jones P, Wilson DM (2010) Network biology as a new approach to drug discovery. Current Opinion in Drug Discovery and Development 13: 524-526

[15] Mostrag-Szlichtyng A, ZaldÃ-var Comenges J-M, Worth AP (2010) Computational toxicology at the European Commission's Joint Research Centre. Expert Opinion on Drug Metabolism & Toxicology 6: 785-792

[16] Muster W, Breidenbach A, Fischer H, Kirchner S, Muller L, Pahler A (2008) Computational toxicology in drug development. Drug Discov Today 13: 303-10

[17] Paul SM, Mytelka DS, Dunwiddie CT, Persinger CC, Munos BH, Lindborg SR, Schacht AL (2010) How to improve R&D productivity: the pharmaceutical industry's grand challenge. Nat Rev Drug Discov 9: 203-214

[18] Rosenfeld S, Kapetanovic I (2008) Systems biology and cancer prevention: all options on the table. Gene Regul Syst Bio 2: 307-19

[19] Roth BL, Sheffler DJ, Kroeze WK (2004) Magic shotguns versus magic bullets: selectively non-selective drugs for mood disorders and schizophrenia. Nat Rev Drug Discov 3: 353-9

[20] Roukos DH (2011) Networks medicine: From reductionism to evidence of complex dynamic biomolecular interactions. Pharmacogenomics 12: 695-698

[21] Sistare FD, Dieterle F, Troth S, Holder DJ, Gerhold D, Andrews-Cleavenger D, Baer W, Betton G, Bounous D, Carl K, Collins N, Goering P, Goodsaid F, Gu YZ, Guilpin V, Harpur E, Hassan A, Jacobson-Kram D, Kasper P, Laurie D, Lima BS, Maciulaitis R, Mattes W, Maurer G, Obert LA, Ozer J, Papaluca-Amati M, Phillips JA, Pinches M, Schipper MJ, Thompson KL, Vamvakas S, Vidal JM, Vonderscher J, Walker E, Webb C, Yu Y (2010) Towards consensus practices to qualify safety biomarkers for use in early drug development. Nat Biotechnol 28: 446-54

[22] Sugiyama Y, Yamashita S (2011) Impact of microdosing clinical study -- Why necessary and how useful? Advanced Drug Delivery Reviews 63: 494-502

[23] van Vliet E (2011) Current Standing and Future Prospects for the Technologies Proposed to Transform Toxicity Testing in the 21(st) Century. Altex-Alternatives to Animal Experimentation 28: 17-44

[24] Wagner JA (2008) Back to the future: driving innovation in drug development. Clin Pharmacol Ther 83: 199-202

Part 1

Current Status and Future Directions

Evolutionary Biology and Drug Development

Pierre M. Durand and Theresa L. Coetzer

University of the Witwatersrand and National Health Laboratory Service

South Africa

1. Introduction

Evolution is the unifying framework in biology and scales to all living systems. It is the central organizing concept to explain seemingly disparate biological phenomena; from the very small (individual molecules) to the very large (ecosystems), from the rise and spread of molecular variants to the behavior and body shapes of elephants. In recent times, our appreciation for evolution in medicine has gained momentum. Individuals have championed the cause, dedicated journals have emerged, and new books on the subject are frequently published ("The Evolution and Medicine Review" is an excellent web-based resource providing updated information on the subject, http://evmedreview.com). This union between evolution and medicine has already advanced our understanding of pathological processes (Maccullum, 2007, Nesse & Stearns, 2008).

Drug development and therapeutic strategies are areas in which evolutionary principles may be particularly helpful. The avalanche of bioinformatic methods, genomic data and subsequent emergence of evolutionary genomics in the last few decades means that integrating these fields in drug design is now a possibility. Incorporating evolutionary information is not only helpful *a posteriori* when we may hope to understand why resistance to a particular compound emerged. It is also valuable *a priori*, to design more efficacious drugs, suggest potential resistance profiles and conceptualize novel treatment strategies. Many allopathic treatments, particularly those for chronic non-infectious diseases, relate to the manipulation of cellular functions within one individual's lifespan, for example, developing a drug aimed at a particular cardiac disorder. In these instances, evolutionary biology may explain why a particular disease arose, the evolutionary relationships between genes in the animal model and human or which pathological processes should be targeted. From an evolutionary perspective populations of reproducing individuals are the material on which evolution acts. Adaptive and non-adaptive changes occur over successive generations, and infectious organisms and cancer are therefore the premier examples to illustrate the role of evolution in drug development. In the current age it is almost unthinkable that evolutionary theory, the only scientific framework for studying ultimate causality in biology, doesn't already form the starting point for developing therapeutic interventions affecting evolving populations.

Here we wish to illustrate the role of evolution in allopathic medicine. A brief overview of the typical drug development pipeline is provided, followed by a discussion of relevant evolutionary questions. We discuss in greater detail the molecular evolutionary processes impacting on the emergence of drug resistance and offer suggestions to limit the problem.

Finally, we discuss the rapidly growing areas of evolvability and multilevel selection and how these inform our understanding of therapeutic strategies.

2. Drug discovery strategies

A drug discovery pipeline is a complex, costly and lengthy process involving several discrete stages (Fig. 1). The median time for the development of a new drug is estimated at ~13 years, with a potential cost upwards of ~1 billion US dollars (Paul et al., 2010). The funnel shape of the pipeline reflects the high failure rate between different stages and fewer than 1 in 50 projects deliver a drug to the market (Brown & Superti-Furga, 2003). In the last few years especially the number of new approved drugs has declined sharply despite an increase in research and development spending. Data from a survey of nine large pharmaceutical companies revealed that in 2010 only two new molecular entities from all these companies were approved by the FDA, a very poor return on their expenditure of approximately $60 billion dollars (Bunnage, 2011). Several strategies have recently been proposed to reduce the costs and improve the success rates, including closer cooperation between pharmaceutical companies and academia (Cressey, 2011, Frye et al., 2011); investigation of new uses for approved drugs (Littman, 2011); increased use of translational phenotypic assays (Swinney & Anthony, 2011); and improved target and lead selection (Brown & Superti-Furga, 2003, Bunnage, 2011).

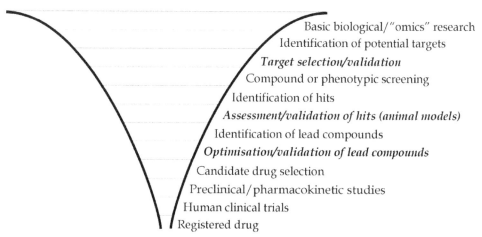

Fig. 1. The drug discovery funnel.

Evolutionary considerations are critical at steps in bold italics.

The availability of whole genome sequences, new discoveries regarding the molecular basis of disease, technological advances in target and lead validation, and high throughput screening strategies, provide exciting opportunities for drug discovery. However, translational research requires improved coordination and integration between different scientific disciplines to ensure a justified transition past key decision points in the drug development pipeline. In this regard, it is critical that evolutionary biologists participate in the process to ensure that fundamental evolutionary principles are taken into account, especially at the validation steps (Fig. 1), to reduce costs and attrition.

3. Evolutionary concepts relevant to drug design

To understand the evolutionary pressures on a potential drug target and the homologous relationships between target genes in the human and the proposed animal model, a few basic concepts should be addressed (Box 1). The reader is referred elsewhere for further discussion of general concepts of molecular evolution (Li, 2006).

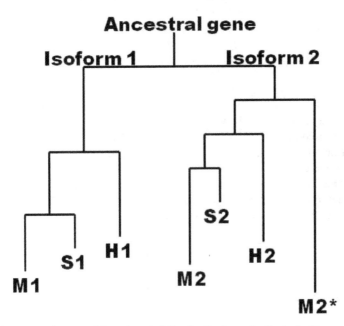

Box 1. Orthology, paralogy and functional shifts. In the hypothetical phylogram an ancestral gene has been duplicated to give paralogous isoforms 1 and 2 in mouse (M), rat (R) and human (H). Speciation events gave rise to orthologues M1, R1 and H1 and orthologues M2, R2 and H2. In the mouse there has been a second duplication event giving rise to M2*. The finding that M2* is isolated on a long branch indicates a functional shift in this gene

3.1 Orthology and paralogy

Homologous genes share a common ancestry and depending on the events in their history are orthologous or paralogous (Box 1). Orthologues arise from speciation events; paralogues arise from gene duplication events and resolving these relationships is best done with phylogenetic reconstructions. A number of methods can be used to re-create phylogeny (Felsenstein, 2004) each with their own strengths and weaknesses, however, it should be borne in mind that phylogenetic reconstructions are not foolproof and may require significant interpretation and re-examination. Processes like concerted evolution, horizontal gene transfer and incongruent evolution cloud the picture (Felsenstein, 2004, Li, 2006). Nevertheless, establishing orthology and paralogy (as best one can) raises major questions and both are important for drug development and assessment of drug targets (Searls, 2003). Orthology informs one about the corresponding gene(s) in the animal model while paralogous relationships are often more important for identifying functional divergence.

3.2 Evolutionary rates

Related to the reconstruction of phylogenetic relationships is the determination of evolutionary rates and patterns. The simplest way of estimating the nature and intensity of the selective pressure is to quantify the ratio of non-synonymous to synonymous nucleotide substitutions in a coding sequence, corrected for opportunity, taking into account various features of sequence evolution such as transition/transversion ratios, base and codon biases, etc (Box 2) (some key references are Goldman & Yang, 1994, Hurst, 2002, Muse & Gaut, 1994, Nei & Gojobori, 1986, Yang, 2006, Yang & Nielsen, 2000). The ratio (dN/dS or ω) reflects fitness advantages or disadvantages resulting from changes in the amino acid sequence. A ratio $\omega>1$ indicates positive (diversifying or adaptive) selection; $\omega<1$ is negative (purifying or stabilizing) selection. In positive selection non-synonymous mutations are more prevalent in extant sequences presumably because they confer a fitness advantage. Negative selection indicates a fitness cost to non-synonymous substitutions. Furthermore, the lower the ω value, the stronger the stabilizing pressure as fewer and fewer non-synonymous substitutions are tolerated. If there is no difference between dN and dS substitution rates ($\omega=1$), the selective pressure is neither stabilizing nor diversifying and evolution is neutral. Examining the evolutionary pressures not only informs one about functional divergence; but guides the researcher in the selection of the target site. Briefly, sites that are fast evolving are typically poor drug targets, while structurally and functionally conserved sites are usually under purifying selection and make more suitable targets.

$$
Q_{ij} = \begin{cases} 0 \\ \Pi_j \\ \kappa\Pi_j \\ \omega\kappa\Pi_j \\ \omega\Pi_j \\ \omega\kappa\Pi_j \end{cases}
$$

Box 2. A model for codon evolution (Goldman & Yang, 1994, Muse & Gaut, 1994). Numerous methods are available to quantify evolutionary rates in nucleotide sequences. An extensively used approach is the maximum likelihood (ML) codon model for evolution. A simplified substitution rate matrix used by the ML method to estimate codon evolution is given (left). The matrix is used to statistically determine evolutionary pressures acting at individual codons: positive, negative or neutral evolution (see text for more discussion and references below). This model determines the probability that codon i mutates to j in a specified time interval and accounts for the transition/transversion rate ratio (κ); the equilibrium frequency of codon j (Π_j); and the non-synonymous/synonymous rate ratio (ω). $Q_{ij} = 0$ if i and j differ at more than 1 position.

4. Evolution and target selection

One of the major causes of attrition of a potential drug candidate is poor quality of the target. The critical steps of target selection and validation require greater emphasis and incorporation of additional evolutionary criteria to reduce subsequent failure.

4.1 Has the target undergone functional divergence?
Many genes of therapeutic interest have undergone expansion leading to functional redundancy. Targeting a specific protein isn't helpful if there are other family members that are immune to the drug and at the same time take over the function of the target.

To assess functional shifts, paralogy is a critical consideration. The reason is pleiotropy, which is often associated with paralogous genes. Pleiotropy occurs when a gene product has more than one function and can either precede gene duplications or result from duplication events where the duplicated gene is less constrained and free to evolve multiple functions. The impact of pleiotropy on drug discovery is apparent when one considers that in these situations, one must disentangle the compound's effect on multiple pathways. A good example of gene duplications leading to pleiotropy and functional divergence is that of the caspase family. The ancestral metazoan caspase has undergone numerous gene duplications over time resulting in at least 11 human and 10 murine true caspase genes (Nedelcu, 2009, Uren *et al.*, 2000, Wang & Gu, 2001). In humans, distinct clusters of caspases have been identified (Uren *et al.*, 2000, Wang & Gu, 2001), which may be involved in evolutionarily related but biochemically distinct pathways of inflammation or apoptosis. It also seems likely that some of the caspase family members are implicated in both processes. These proteins are primarily involved in one of the processes but are pleiotropically linked to the other. Disentangling the role of individual caspases in the two pathways would be important for developing drugs targeting either inflammation or apoptosis.

5. Evolution and hit validation

The assessment of hit compounds often requires *in vivo* testing in animal models and an inappropriate choice of model is one of the reasons why an apparently promising lead compound fails during human clinical trials. Understanding the phylogenetic relationships between genes in the two systems is therefore an important initial step.

5.1 What are the evolutionary relationships between genes in the model and target organisms?
The biochemical and pharmacological findings in an experimental model organism cannot be extrapolated to another organism without understanding the evolutionary relationships between the target genes. This is because evolutionary rates and functional divergence between homologous genes in related organisms may vary. It is important; therefore, to establish at the very least the homologous relationships between the gene used in the experimental system and the proposed target gene in the human.

Even a slightly improved understanding of orthologous gene differences between model and target species can have an impact on the progression of a compound with major implications for scientific and financial resources. However, while orthology tells us about the evolutionary relationships between genes in related organisms and *suggests* similar function, this is not guaranteed. A phylogram may reveal that a particular gene in the model organism is orthologous to the gene in the target organism. Despite this orthologous relationship isolation of the gene on its own long branch indicates sequence divergence and a functional shift. This should alert the researcher to be wary of using that particular model as a basis for studying the biochemistry of the protein in the human target. In the example given in Box 1 a duplication event has led to genes M2 and M2* in the mouse. This duplication occurred after the speciation events giving rise to humans and rats and both M2 and M2* are therefore orthologues of R2 and H2. However, the isolation of M2* on its own long branch strongly suggests functional divergence and it should not be used as a model for developing a drug compound targeted at H2.

Molecular evolution of homologous proteins may vary along different lineages, which means that a protein may appear highly stable and conserved in one branch leading to humans, but under a different selective pressure in the experimental model animal. If this is not taken into account inappropriate models may be selected. A good example of this is the finding that leptin is associated with obesity in mice (Chen *et al.*, 1996). The discovery was greeted with tremendous excitement since it implied that rodents could be used as a model organism for studying the pathogenesis of obesity in humans. However, it subsequently emerged that there is evidence for positive selection in leptin in primates (including humans) but not in rodents (Benner *et al.*, 2000). This indicates adaptive evolution and a functional shift in leptin after the divergence of primates from rodents. Using the mouse therefore, as a model for understanding the biochemistry of the protein and its potential use as a drug target in humans is problematic.

6. Harnessing evolution to minimize the emergence of resistance

Drug resistance is an ever present threat that curtails the effective lifespan of a drug and has enormous financial implications for pharmaceutical companies. Resistance can develop very rapidly, for example, resistance to the anti-malaria drugs pyrimethamine and proguanil (Hyde, 2005) developed within a year of introducing the drug to the market. Similarly, chronic myeloid leukaemia (CML) cells have become refractory to treatment with tyrosine kinase inhibitors targeting the bcr-abl oncogenic protein, necessitating the development of second and third generation inhibitors (Kantarjian *et al.*, 2008). It is therefore vital that evolutionary principles are applied to the key decision points in the drug development process relating to the validation of targets, hits and lead compounds to minimize the emergence of resistance.

6.1 What is the possible evolutionary response to drug pressure?

Evolution occurs by non-adaptive and adaptive (Darwinian) means. Non-adaptive evolution includes pleiotropic phenomena and genetic drift, or may appear non-adaptive at one level of selection and adaptive at another. Adaptive evolution occurs by natural selection and is more closely associated with the concept of fitness. For pharmacological interventions against infections and cancer to be effective, they are aimed at killing or at least inhibiting growth of infective organisms or cancer cells. This means they generally act on adaptive traits so that fitness is compromised. Targeting a non-adaptive trait such as the pleiotropic effects of paralogous genes discussed above may have a minimal effect on fitness, limiting the drug's usefulness. Targeting fitness-related traits is important for a drug to be effective, but doing so induces a Darwinian response if there are any survivors following the treatment. Furthermore, the greater the fitness cost resulting from the drug pressure the stronger the evolutionary response (Read *et al.*, 2011), and it is usually a question of *when*, rather than *if*, resistant mutants will emerge.

There is effectively a therapeutic trade-off. From the perspective of treatment efficacy, the trade-off is between maximizing the fitness cost to the target (infectious agent or cancer cell) and minimizing the undesirable evolutionary escape response. Of course, if the fitness cost is absolute and all individuals in the population of infective organisms or cancer cells are killed, there is no trade-off. This is the ideal situation; but often not the case. Unless there is complete cure, there will be a therapeutic trade-off. Optimizing this trade-off is seldom given any consideration and therapy results in a temporary hiatus in the disease. Eventually the most resistant mutants take over and, as indicated, the most aggressive therapies elicit the strongest escape response (Read *et al.*, 2011). In addition, not only does therapy select the most virulent individuals, but the group level dynamic is disrupted, further intensifying the escape response. Studies in mice infected with the malaria parasite *Plasmodium chabaudi* found that more virulent clones are controlled by less virulent ones (Wargo *et al.*, 2007). Treatment that failed to eradicate all clones allowed the more virulent ones to thrive leading to a more serious secondary relapse. Humans living in malaria endemic areas can be infected with over 15 genotypically distinct clones of *P. falciparum* (Juliano *et al.*, 2010). If the mouse model study is extrapolated to humans, then aggressive chemotherapy may actually be harmful in the long-term. Instead, to optimize the therapeutic trade-off, it is suggested that the guiding principle should be to impose no more selection than is absolutely necessary (Read *et al.*, 2011). This holds particular relevance for infections or malignancies where cure is unlikely and therapy is aimed more at disease management, for example, chronic leukaemias and infections like HIV.

An understanding of the evolutionary constraints acting at the molecular level is not only helpful when predicting the intensity of the evolutionary response, but it is also important for identifying the appropriate target sites of a protein.

6.2 Can we identify target sites with minimal risk for resistance?

There are various computational approaches (see Yang, 1997 and later versions) to determine the selective pressures acting on whole genes, specific codons or on lineages in a phylogenetic tree. Whole genes are seldom under positive selection; however, those that are, rapidly escape the fitness cost associated with the drug therapy. Non-synonymous substitutions already confer a fitness advantage in sequences demonstrating positive selection and the added drug pressure rapidly leads to resistance. To obtain a more informative view of a gene's evolutionary rate, it is helpful to examine substitution rates at individual codons in the coding sequence. Maximum likelihood estimates of ω at individual codons will usually reveal variation across the coding sequence. Highly conserved or functionally important amino acids are likely to be under purifying selection, while others in the sequence may be evolving neutrally or be under positive selection. Targeting the positively selected or neutral sites will drive the emergence of resistance mutations and should be avoided, while sites under intense purifying selective pressures are far less likely to produce viable mutations and make suitable targets.

Drug treatments add to the naturally occurring selective pressures and codon sites that code for resistant mutations are frequently evolving more rapidly than others. A good example of this is a study of serially sampled reverse transcriptase coding sequences isolated from a group of HIV-1 subtype C–infected women before and after single-dose nevirapine (Seoighe *et al.*, 2007). Nevirapine is a standard therapy for preventing mother-to-child transmission. A directional selection evolutionary model differentiated codons under positive selection from those subject to purifying selection and the differences in evolutionary rates would reliably have predicted *a priori* the sites of amino acid change leading to nevirapine resistance. This study provided proof of concept that quantifying the evolutionary pressures acting at individual codon sites can predict the likelihood of resistance emerging if the drug-protein binding site is known. Even before this study, others developed iterative approaches for use in development pipelines to guide experimentalists to biologically relevant sites based on sequence conservation. The first approach known as Evolutionary Tracing (ET) (Lichtarge *et al.*, 1996, Lichtarge & Sowa, 2002) and another, Evolutionary Patterning (EP) (Durand *et al.*, 2008), which directly quantifies the evolutionary rate, provide useful examples for further illustration.

6.2.1 Evolutionary tracing

ET generates a trace sequence from multiple sequence alignments of functional classes of a protein family. Clusters of invariant amino acids are identified and incorporated into 3D structures to identify the most suitable target sites in terms of their conservation, functional and structural importance and access. ET is particularly helpful for modeling functional specificity and architecture-defining residues. ET predictions have been verified experimentally. The most complete demonstration that ET anticipates mutational and crystallographic analyses was performed on the regulator of G protein signaling proteins that act to increase G_α GTP hydrolysis rates (Sowa *et al.*, 2000). Based on the ET data specific amino acids were mutated causing profound effects on enzyme activity and led to the prediction of an allosteric binding site (Sowa *et al.*, 2001), which was subsequently confirmed by crystallography (Slep *et al.*, 2001).

6.2.2 Evolutionary patterning

In ET, one of the premises for identifying target sites is that structurally and functionally essential amino acids are conserved in a trace sequence. However, while conservation suggests purifying selection it does not necessarily equate to it. To more accurately quantify the selective pressure acting at a particular amino acid residue, it is important to study the substitution rates at individual codons across a coding sequence. This is the approach adopted by EP, which makes use of a maximum likelihood substitution matrix to estimate the ratio of non-synonymous / synonymous substitutions at individual codons in a coding sequence (Box 2). The Bayes Empirical Bayes posterior probability of the MLE (maximum likelihood estimate) of ω falling into a particular category (for example, positive selection $\omega > 1$ or extreme purifying selection $\omega < 0.1$) is computed using PAML software (Yang, 2007). The distribution of these probabilities across a potential target protein can be examined and mapped to the predicted 3D structure, guiding the researcher as to which residues to target and which to avoid. It is argued that codons subject to extreme purifying selection are evolutionarily constrained, perhaps because the amino acid is essential for protein structure or function. The data from extant sequences indicate that non-synonymous mutations at these sites are not tolerated and make ideal drug targets if the encoded amino acids are accessible to interactions with lead compounds. In contrast, residues that are subject to positive or neutral selection, or only weakly conserved should be avoided. Non-synonymous mutations at these sites have arisen naturally during the evolutionary history of the protein indicating that amino acid changes do not significantly compromise protein fitness. These sites should not be targeted therapeutically as any mutants that arise are likely to be selected for by the drug pressure. Mapping the amino acids under extreme purifying selection to a structural model is important so that the accessibility and interaction between target sites and lead compounds can be assessed *in silico*. As with ET, this is an iterative process. Docking studies uncover drug-protein interactions and the strength of chemical bonds assessed; interactions with undesirable amino acids are revealed and the lead compound may be modified so that contacts with target sites are optimized. The process can then be repeated as often as necessary to maximize favourable interactions.

The application of EP to a potential drug target, *P. falciparum* glycerol kinase may be used as an illustration (Figures 2 and 3) (Durand *et al.*, 2008). Six separate target sites comprising stretches of contiguous amino acids subject to extreme purifying selection were identified. The targets were mapped to a 3D model generated using the *E. coli* homologue as a template, which revealed that four were accessible to potential lead compounds. These sites were also found to overlap with functional domains and were suggested as therapeutic targets. The EP approach was validated by examining resistance mutations in the *P. falciparum* dihydrofolate reductase-thymidylate synthase protein, which is targeted by the anti-malarial drug pyrimethamine. EP predicted that none of the five known mutations conferring pyrimethamine resistance would have been subject to extreme purifying selection - a factor which would have facilitated the evolution of resistance. This was indeed the case, confirming that the likelihood of an evolutionary escape response was greater if the codon was under more relaxed evolutionary constraints.

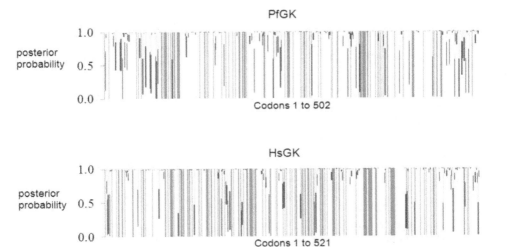

Fig. 2. Posterior probabilities for four categories of ω across GK coding sequences (from Durand *et al.*, 2008). Bayes Empirical Bayes posterior probability estimates for each category of ω across *P. falciparum* (PfGK) and human (HsGK) GK coding sequences are shown. Residues under extreme purifying selection (ω≤0.1) are potential drug target sites and were mapped to a 3D model to assess drug accessibility (Fig. 3). Categories for ω are indicated with coloured bars: yellow (ω>1.0), red (ω=1.0), white (0.1<ω<1.0), and blue (ω≤0.1).

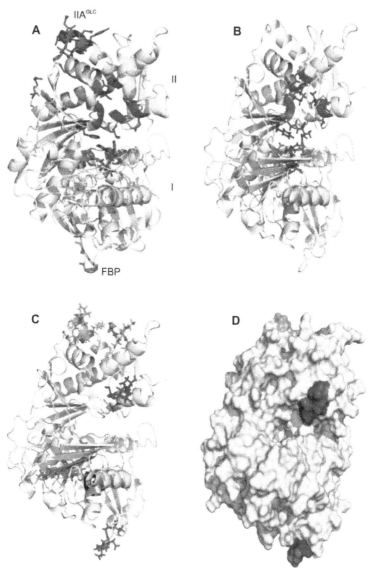

Fig. 3. *E. coli* and *P. falciparum* glycerol kinase 3D models (from Durand *et al.*, 2008). Ribbon models (with functional residues as sticks) of E. coli glycerol kinase (EcGK) (A) and P. falciparum glycerol kinase (PfGK) (B) are displayed. In EcGK, coloured residues are involved in binding to ADP (blue), Mg2+ (yellow), glycerol (red), FBP (fructose-bis-phosphate) (orange) and IIAGLC (purple).   Alpha helices and ß sheets in the ATPase site (light green) and subunit interactions (aquamarine) are shown. The PfGK model is based on EcGK. Five regions were identified in Fig. 2 as good target sites and mapped to ribbon (C) and surface (D) models. One of the regions (black) is partly obscured and is in the core of the molecule, indicating the region would not be accessible to drug compounds.

ET and EP provide guidance for selecting the most suitable drug target sites and thus assist in designing more effective drugs, which may limit the emergence of resistance for long periods. However, any drug pressure will still invoke an evolutionary response, so at some point escape mutants are still likely to arise. A truly fundamental shift in the approach to allopathic therapies would involve strategies aimed at having evolution work in our favour rather than against us. Doing so is a major conceptual challenge.

7. Evolvability and multilevel selection: Future avenues for drug research

Basic science research into the fundamental nature of evolution has resulted in what some biologists think is tantamount to a paradigm shift. For a review of these advances see discussions around an "extended theory of evolution" (Danchin et al., 2011). Two areas in which evolutionary thinking has rapidly progressed are the concepts of evolvability and multilevel selection. Both have relevance for future drug development strategies.

7.1 Evolvability

Advances in evolution hold promise for exploiting under-appreciated biological phenomena in drug design. The eloquent statement "Not only has life evolved, but life has evolved to evolve" (Earl & Deem, 2004) implies that the genetically encoded propensity to adapt to environmental pressures (known as evolvability) is a selectable phenotype. The variation in response to changing environments confers heritable variation in fitness. It is argued therefore, that evolvability can be acted on by natural selection leading to populations of organisms that are more or less likely to adapt to environmental pressures. Experimental evolution studies using model organisms like *Escherichia* (Leroi et al., 1994) and *Chlamydomonas* (Bell & Reboud, 1997) date back nearly two decades and seem to support these assertions although whether evolvability itself is always adaptive (as opposed to being non-adaptive) is not always clear (Creavin, 2004). Evolvability also appears to play a role in pathogen virulence. For example, the HIV reverse transcriptase (RT) is notoriously error-prone leading to the evolution of populations of quasispecies that evade host immunity and escape drug pressures (Bebenek et al., 1993). However, as indicated above, whether the error prone nature of HIV RT evolved as an adaptation or whether it is the result of other adaptive or non-adaptive effects is uncertain. Nevertheless, what is clear is that the error rate of HIV RT confers a fitness advantage. Targeting the pathogen's evolvability rather than phenotypic traits that are easily overcome by the propensity to evolve is therefore likely to have a greater impact in the long term. It can be argued that where evolvability forms part of a pathogen's life history strategy, this consideration should be included in drug design efforts. For further discussion on plasticity and evolvability in parasitic infections such as malaria with relevance to chemotherapeutic strategies the reader is referred elsewhere (for example Reece et al., 2009).

7.2 Multilevel selection theory
7.2.1 Multilevel selection, sociobiology and the conceptualization of novel drug strategies

Our understanding of the living world has been transformed by the finding that natural selection acts at multiple levels of biological organization (Box 3). Multilevel selection theory (MLST), which includes group selection and for which there is now a significant body of evidence, describes the living world in terms of hierarchically structured levels where the tenets of selection are applicable to evolutionary units across these levels (Keller, 1999, Lewontin, 1970, Okasha, 2006, Wilson, 1975). Evolutionary transitions gave rise to increasing complexity including groups of genes, which form genomes, which form cells, which form multicellular organisms, which may form social groups and so on (Maynard Smith & Száthmary, 1995). The fact that the units of evolution span levels of biological organization raises the question of whether it may be better to target other levels of organization such as groups rather than individual cancer cells or infectious organisms.

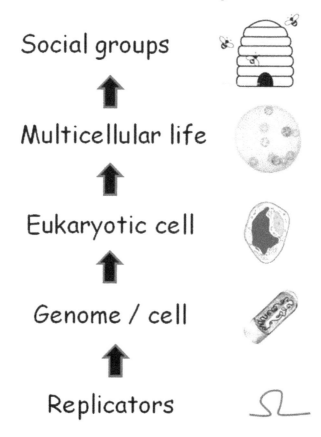

Social groups

⬆

Multicellular life

⬆

Eukaryotic cell

⬆

Genome / cell

⬆

Replicators

Box 3. The multilevel selection paradigm. The living world is characterized by quantum leaps in organization and complexity. Early replicators cooperated to form genomes and cells, which formed a eukaryotic cell, multicellular life, social groups and so on. Evolution by natural selection acts on any system where there is a group of reproducing individuals, so long as there is heritable variation in fitness. All these levels are therefore subject to natural selection. The related concept of group selection fits into this framework of MLST and describes competition between rather than within groups. While there is ongoing debate regarding the mechanisms, terminology and extent of group selection most researchers accept the fundamentals.

For drug development strategists, there are some key aspects to MLST that must be appreciated. Group level traits and adaptations arise because of selection and dynamics between groups rather than individuals within a group. These traits arise in various ways. They can be aggregates of properties within the group or arise as irreducible 'emergent properties' only existing at the group level (Thompson, 2000). Selection pressures at different levels of organization can vary; a particular trait can be beneficial at one level and harmful at another (see programmed cell death later) or the trait may have differential fitness benefits at two or more levels. Unpacking the relative selection pressures at different levels requires an understanding of Fisher's fundamental theorem of natural selection, which states that "*the rate of increase in fitness of any organism at any time is equal to its genetic variance in fitness at that time*" (Fisher, 1930). Fisher's theorem is applicable at any level of organization, whether it is a population of groups or a population of cells. Drugs targeting more than one level of selection will therefore induce differential responses and the intensity of the evolutionary escape response will depend on fitness variances at the different levels. Targeting the group level, rather than individuals as is the conventional approach has distinct advantages for therapies against infections (Pepper, 2008) and cancer (Pepper et al., 2009). The advantages typically concern the phenomenon of cooperation and the group fitness variance.

The phenomena of cooperation and its more extreme form altruism are commonly found in groups of pathogens or cancer cells. Mechanistically, cooperation can take the form of "public goods" (Wessler et al., 2007), molecules that are produced by individuals but have a group level action. The quantity or quality of molecule produced by one of the individuals is of such a nature that it may have little or no direct benefit for the producer, but in combination with the molecular products from others results in a group level fitness-enhancing trait. For example, in bacterial biofilms quorum-sensing molecules regulate cell division of individuals so that the group responds to challenges as a collective (Wessler et al., 2007). Similarly, in solid tumours angiogenic factors are produced by individual cells but only when sufficient quantities are produced by the group does neo-vascularization occur (Kerbel, 1991). Targeting public goods makes good evolutionary sense.

Consider a situation where individuals (cancer cells or pathogens) secrete molecules that only have a group level benefit. There is initially no benefit for a mutant individual because the concentration of its molecular product is either too low or on its own cannot modify the group phenotype and increase group fitness. More likely, its mutant nature means that its role in the group network is compromised and group fitness is diminished. Unlike conventional therapies which actively select for resistance, there is no immediate fitness benefit to mutants and resistant individuals die along with others in the group or they are selected against. Of course, a larger clone of resistant cells may survive and reproduce, but from the outset and all else being equal, mutants have the same or lower fitness than susceptible cells and generally do not take over the population. This scenario is more than just conceptual. It is supported empirically. One of the most detailed illustrations comes from the 15 year old study of tumour neo-vascularization and drug resistance referred to above (Boehm et al., 1997, Kerbel, 1991).

In solid tumours cancer cells eventually outgrow their nutrient supply. Angiogenesis factors are produced by the tumour leading to neo-vascularization and subsequent survival of the group. Cytotoxic cancer drugs create a powerful selective pressure and in the heterogeneous population of cancer cells resistance rapidly emerges. However, targeting the group level benefit with "anti-angiogenic therapy does not induce drug resistance" (Boehm et al., 1997).

This is because while the angiogenesis blocker is applied, resistant mutants do not produce sufficient angiogenesis factors for neo-vascularization to occur and they die along with others before reaching a critical mass.

Similar strategies have been advocated or used for a number of infectious diseases with some success, including the escalating challenge of methicillin-resistant *S. aureus* (MRSA) (see Pepper, 2008 and references therein). *S. aureus* produces numerous virulence molecules that act at the group level and are required for establishing and maintaining infections. The prototypical public good example in *S aureus* is α–toxin, without which infections in animal models are unsustainable (Bhakdi & Tranum-Jensen, 1991). A literature survey suggests that an appropriate and current opportunity for using MLST in drug development is tuberculosis (TB). TB is one of the major global health challenges and with the emergence of multidrug resistant (MDR) and extreme drug resistant (XDR) strains the need for novel strategies has never been more urgent. Laboratory studies of the resuscitation promoting factors (rpfs) in *Mycobacterium* species indicate that these factors may be prime targets for group level chemotherapy (for a review of rpfs see Kana & Mizrahi, 2010). Knockout experiments suggest rpfs have a negligible role in individual cell fitness; however, at the group level they are important as virulence factors and for the resuscitation of latent infections.

With regards to fitness variance and the rate of evolution, Fisher's theorem bodes well for drug strategies targeting cooperation in groups. The fitness variance of the phenotype decreases as the cooperative behaviour increases and is shared equally within the group (for a detailed discussion see Price, 1972). When fitness variance is zero, the implication is that either all the individuals in the group receive the benefit of the public good or none at all. The evolutionary rate of the group level phenotype is therefore exceedingly slow, as is the likelihood of resistance developing. This is in contrast to the evolutionary rates when the unit of selection is the individual in the group. In these instances fitness variance is usually greater and resistance evolves more rapidly. The fundamental properties of evolutionary rates as they relate to fitness variance coupled with cooperation and group level traits opens a whole new avenue for drug development strategies.

7.2.2 Multilevel selection and the intriguing case of programmed cell death

The phenomenon of programmed cell death (PCD) in unicellular eukaryotes brings together many aspects discussed in this chapter. It provides a useful context for integrating homology, adaptations, evolutionary rates, evolvability and MLST as they relate to infections, cancer and drug development. Our discussion of PCD below is based on a few key papers and requires far more investigation, but as an example it illustrates how evolutionary thinking could lead to a radical shift in drug design.

Programmed cell death (PCD), previously considered a hallmark of multicellularity, has been reported in all major lineages in unicellular eukaryotes and prokaryotes (see Table 1 in Nedelcu *et al.*, 2011). From an evolutionary perspective (with implications for drug design in infections and cancer) the burning question has been: why would an organism actively kill itself? For an individual unicellular organism PCD has no fitness benefit and adaptive evolution cannot explain the phenomenon. Likely explanations are that it is either maladaptive pleiotropy or adaptive in a MLS context (i.e. at a group level). While strong arguments can be made for both scenarios (Nedelcu *et al.*, 2011), laboratory evidence from two model organisms favour the hypothesis that PCD in unicells is adaptive for the group. In *S. cerevisiae* PCD-related aging assists re-growth in a related mutant subpopulation

(Fabrizio *et al.*, 2004, Herker *et al.*, 2004). A direct fitness-related experiment in *C. reinhardtii* demonstrated that molecules released by cells dying by PCD provide fitness benefits to others (Durand *et al.*, 2011). Genomic studies have also revealed that many of the homologues for key protein domains involved in PCD are conserved across a wide range of organisms (for example Nedelcu, 2009), although there has been expansion of many of the gene families, particularly in vertebrates and plants as organism complexity evolved. As discussed in sections 3 and 4, an understanding of the evolutionary rates and relationships between homologues in model and target organisms will be helpful if expanded gene families in the PCD pathway are to be targeted therapeutically.

S. cerevisiae and *C. reinhardtii* are already used as model organisms for a range of diseases including cancer (for example Fang & Umen, 2008). The genomic and empirical data for PCD as an adaptation in these organisms shed new light on PCD in human parasitic infections and cancer and can help explain some puzzling phenomena. With regards to parasitic disease, numerous organisms demonstrate PCD, including apicomplexa, stramenopiles, trichomonads, diplomonads, kinetoplastids and trypanosomatids (see Table 1 in Nedelcu *et al.*, 2011 and references therein). The group effect of PCD in most of these organisms has not been studied; however, in *Leishmania* (a kinetoplastid) infections, PCD as a group level adaptation explains the counterintuitive finding that virulence is associated with PCD (Van Zandbergen *et al.*, 2006). If the infective inoculum contains a proportion of apoptotic (PCD) cells, the population has greater virulence and fitness. Removing the apoptotic forms diminishes disease severity. The interpretation is that apoptotic forms enhance group fitness, which is in keeping with the *C. reinhardtii* findings. Similar experiments have not been performed with cancer cells, but the role of apoptosis is not always clear. Tumour suppressor genes are usually mutated in cancer; however, the apoptosis pathway is malignant cells is frequently activated through the FAS ligand receptor. Curiously, the FAS ligand pathway can also promote tumour growth (Chen *et al.*, 2010). Whether this is due to crosstalk between this pathway and another anti-apoptosis pathway is unclear. However, in light of the *C. reinhardtii* experiments (Durand *et al.*, 2011) and that the essential pathology of cancer is atavism (regression to the ancestral unicellular state) (Davies & Lineweaver), is it possible that apoptosis in some cancers also provides benefits to other cells in the population? In a bizarre twist, can chemotherapy exacerbate a cancer or infection by inducing PCD in some cells, which then provide fitness benefits to others?

8. Concluding remarks

The potential role for evolutionary biology in drug design is vast and can be applied at various stages in the development process. The aim here is to provide the reader with an overview of evolutionary medicine, with specific reference to drug design and the emergence of resistance in infections and cancer. Some key concepts such as phylogenetic relationships and evolutionary rates are introduced to illustrate how evolutionary studies can predict the most suitable drug target sites in a protein and limit resistance. Perhaps the most exciting union between evolution and drug development is the future use of evolvability and multilevel selection, heralding a new era for therapeutic strategies.

9. References

Bebenek, K., Abbotts, J., Wilson, S.H. & Kunkel, T.A. (1993) Error-prone polymerization by HIV-1 reverse transcriptase. Contribution of template-primer misalignment, miscoding, and termination probability to mutational hot spots. *J Biol Chem*, 268, 10324-34.

Bell, G. & Reboud, X. (1997) Experimental evolution in Chlamydomonas II. Genetic variation in strongly contrasted environments. *Heredity*, 78, 498-506.

Benner, S.A., Chamberlin, S.G., Liberles, D.A., Govindarajan, S. & Knecht, L. (2000) Functional inferences from reconstructed evolutionary biology involving rectified databases--an evolutionarily grounded approach to functional genomics. *Res Microbiol*, 151, 97-106.

Bhakdi, S. & Tranum-Jensen, J. (1991) Alpha-toxin of Staphylococcus aureus. *Microbiol Rev*, 55, 733-51.

Boehm, T., Folkman, J., Browder, T. & O'Reilly, M.S. (1997) Antiangiogenic therapy of experimental cancer does not induce acquired drug resistance. *Nature*, 390, 404-7.

Brown, D. & Superti-Furga, G. (2003) Rediscovering the sweet spot in drug discovery. *Drug Discov Today*, 8, 1067-77.

Bunnage, M.E. (2011) Getting pharmaceutical R&D back on target. *Nat Chem Biol*, 7, 335-9.

Chen, H., Charlat, O., Tartaglia, L.A., Woolf, E.A., Weng, X., Ellis, S.J., Lakey, N.D., Culpepper, J., Moore, K.J., Breitbart, R.E., Duyk, G.M., Tepper, R.I. & Morgenstern, J.P. (1996) Evidence that the diabetes gene encodes the leptin receptor: identification of a mutation in the leptin receptor gene in db/db mice. *Cell*, 84, 491-5.

Chen, L., Park, S.M., Tumanov, A.V., Hau, A., Sawada, K., Feig, C., Turner, J.R., Fu, Y.X., Romero, I.L., Lengyel, E. & Peter, M.E. (2010) CD95 promotes tumour growth. *Nature*, 465, 492-6.

Creavin, T. (2004) Evolvability: Implications for drug design. *Drug Discov Today*, 3, 178.

Cressey, D. (2011) Traditional drug-discovery model ripe for reform. *Nature*, 471, 17-8.

Danchin, E., Charmantier, A., Champagne, F.A., Mesoudi, A., Pujol, B. & Blanchet, S. (2011) Beyond DNA: integrating inclusive inheritance into an extended theory of evolution. *Nat Rev Genet*, 12, 475-86.

Davies, P.C. & Lineweaver, C.H. Cancer tumors as Metazoa 1.0: tapping genes of ancient ancestors. *Phys Biol*, 8, 015001.

Durand, P.M., Naidoo, K. & Coetzer, T.L. (2008) Evolutionary patterning: a novel approach to the identification of potential drug target sites in Plasmodium falciparum. *PLoS One*, 3, e3685.

Durand, P.M., Rashidi, A. & Michod, R.E. (2011) How an organism dies affects the fitness of its neighbors. *Am Nat*, 177, 224-32.

Earl, D.J. & Deem, M.W. (2004) Evolvability is a selectable trait. *Proc Natl Acad Sci U S A*, 101, 11531-6.

Fabrizio, P., Battistella, L., Vardavas, R., Gattazzo, C., Liou, L.L., Diaspro, A., Dossen, J.W., Gralla, E.B. & Longo, V.D. (2004) Superoxide is a mediator of an altruistic aging program in Saccharomyces cerevisiae. *J Cell Biol*, 166, 1055-67.

Fang, S.C. & Umen, J.G. (2008) A suppressor screen in chlamydomonas identifies novel components of the retinoblastoma tumor suppressor pathway. *Genetics*, 178, 1295-310.

Felsenstein, J. (2004) *Inferring phylogenies*. Sinauer Ass, ISBN 087893775, Sunderland.

Fisher, R.A. (1930) *The genetical theory of natural selection*. Clarendon Press, Oxford.

Frye, S., Crosby, M., Edwards, T. & Juliano, R. (2011) US academic drug discovery. *Nat Rev Drug Discov*, 10, 409-10.

Goldman, N. & Yang, Z. (1994) A codon-based model of nucleotide substitution for protein-coding DNA sequences. *Mol Biol Evol*, 11, 725-36.

Herker, E., Jungwirth, H., Lehmann, K.A., Maldener, C., Frohlich, K.U., Wissing, S., Buttner, S., Fehr, M., Sigrist, S. & Madeo, F. (2004) Chronological aging leads to apoptosis in yeast. *J Cell Biol*, 164, 501-7.

Hurst, L.D. (2002) The Ka/Ks ratio: diagnosing the form of sequence evolution. *Trends Genet*, 18, 486.

Hyde, J.E. (2005) Drug-resistant malaria. *Trends Parasitol*, 21, 494-8.

Juliano, J.J., Porter, K., Mwapasa, V., Sem, R., Rogers, W.O., Ariey, F., Wongsrichanalai, C., Read, A. & Meshnick, S.R. (2010) Exposing malaria in-host diversity and estimating population diversity by capture-recapture using massively parallel pyrosequencing. *Proc Natl Acad Sci U S A*, 107, 20138-43.

Kana, B.D. & Mizrahi, V. (2010) Resuscitation promoting factors in bacterial population dynamics during TB infection *Drug Discov Today*, 7, e13-e18.

Kantarjian, H., Schiffer, C., Jones, D. & Cortes, J. (2008) Monitoring the response and course of chronic myeloid leukemia in the modern era of BCR-ABL tyrosine kinase inhibitors: practical advice on the use and interpretation of monitoring methods. *Blood*, 111, 1774-80.

Keller, L.K. (1999) *Levels of selection in evolution.* Princeton University Press, Princeton, NJ.

Kerbel, R.S. (1991) Inhibition of tumor angiogenesis as a strategy to circumvent acquired resistance to anti-cancer therapeutic agents. *Bioessays*, 13, 31-6.

Leroi, A.M., Bennett, A.F. & Lenski, R.E. (1994) Temperature acclimation and competitive fitness: an experimental test of the beneficial acclimation assumption. *Proc Natl Acad Sci U S A*, 91, 1917-21.

Lewontin, R.C. (1970) The units of selection. *Annu Rev Ecol Syst*, 1, 1-18.

Li, W.H. (2006) *Molecular evolution.* Sinauer Press, ISBN 0878934804, Sunderland.

Lichtarge, O., Bourne, H.R. & Cohen, F.E. (1996) An evolutionary trace method defines binding surfaces common to protein families. *J Mol Biol*, 257, 342-58.

Lichtarge, O. & Sowa, M.E. (2002) Evolutionary predictions of binding surfaces and interactions. *Curr Opin Struct Biol*, 12, 21-7.

Littman, B.H. (2011) An audience with Francis Collins. *Nature Rev Drug Discov*, 10, 14.

MacCullum, C.J. (2007) Does medicine without evolution make sense? *PLoS Biology*, 5, 679-680.

Maynard Smith, J. & Száthmary, E. (1995) *The major transitions in evolution.* W. H. Freeman, ISBN 019850294X, San Francisco.

Muse, S.V. & Gaut, B.S. (1994) A likelihood approach for comparing synonymous and nonsynonymous nucleotide substitution rates, with application to the chloroplast genome. *Mol Biol Evol*, 11, 715-24.

Nedelcu, A.M. (2009) Comparative genomics of phylogenetically diverse unicellular eukaryotes provide new insights into the genetic basis for the evolution of the programmed cell death machinery. *J Mol Evol*, 68, 256-68.

Nedelcu, A.M., Driscoll, W.W., Durand, P.M., Herron, M.D. & Rashidi, A. (2011) On the paradigm of altruistic suicide in the unicellular world. *Evolution*, 65, 3-20.

Nei, M. & Gojobori, T. (1986) Simple methods for estimating the numbers of synonymous and nonsynonymous nucleotide substitutions. *Mol Biol Evol*, 3, 418-26.

Nesse, R.M. & Stearns, S.C. (2008) The great opportunity: Evolutionary applications to medicine and public health. *Evol Appl*, 1, 28-48.

Okasha, S. (2006) *Evolution and the levels of selection.* Oxford University Press, ISBN 9780199267972, New York.

Paul, S.M., Mytelka, D.S., Dunwiddie, C.T., Persinger, C.C., Munos, B.H., Lindborg, S.R. & Schacht, A.L. (2010) How to improve R&D productivity: the pharmaceutical industry's grand challenge. *Nat Rev Drug Discov*, 9, 203-14.

Pepper, J.W. (2008) Defeating pathogen drug resistance: guidance from evolutionary theory. *Evolution*, 62, 3185-91.

Pepper, J.W., Scott Findlay, C., Kassen, R., Spencer, S.L. & Maley, C.C. (2009) Cancer research meets evolutionary biology. *Evol Appl*, 2, 62-70.

Price, G.R. (1972) Fisher's 'fundamental theorem' made clear. *Ann Hum Genet*, 36, 129-40.

Read, A.F., Day, T. & Huijben, S. (2011) Colloquium Paper: The evolution of drug resistance and the curious orthodoxy of aggressive chemotherapy. *Proc Natl Acad Sci U S A*, 108 Suppl 2, 10871-7.

Reece, S.E., Ramiro, R.S. & Nussey, D.H. (2009) Plastic parasites: sophisticated strategies for survival and reproduction? *Evol Appl*, 2, 11-23.

Searls, D.B. (2003) Pharmacophylogenomics: genes, evolution and drug targets. *Nat Rev Drug Discov*, 2, 613-23.

Seoighe, C., Ketwaroo, F., Pillay, V., Scheffler, K., Wood, N., Duffet, R., Zvelebil, M., Martinson, N., McIntyre, J., Morris, L. & Hide, W. (2007) A model of directional selection applied to the evolution of drug resistance in HIV-1. *Mol Biol Evol*, 24, 1025-31.

Slep, K.C., Kercher, M.A., He, W., Cowan, C.W., Wensel, T.G. & Sigler, P.B. (2001) Structural determinants for regulation of phosphodiesterase by a G protein at 2.0 A. *Nature*, 409, 1071-7.

Sowa, M.E., He, W., Slep, K.C., Kercher, M.A., Lichtarge, O. & Wensel, T.G. (2001) Prediction and confirmation of a site critical for effector regulation of RGS domain activity. *Nat Struct Biol*, 8, 234-7.

Sowa, M.E., He, W., Wensel, T.G. & Lichtarge, O. (2000) A regulator of G protein signaling interaction surface linked to effector specificity. *Proc Natl Acad Sci U S A*, 97, 1483-8.

Swinney, D.C. & Anthony, J. (2011) How were new medicines discovered? *Nat Rev Drug Discov*, 10, 507-19.

Thompson, N.S. (2000) Shifting the natural selection metaphor to the group level. *Behavior and Philosophy*, 28, 83-101.

Uren, A.G., O'Rourke, K., Aravind, L.A., Pisabarro, M.T., Seshagiri, S., Koonin, E.V. & Dixit, V.M. (2000) Identification of paracaspases and metacaspases: two ancient families of caspase-like proteins, one of which plays a key role in MALT lymphoma. *Mol Cell*, 6, 961-7.

van Zandbergen, G., Bollinger, A., Wenzel, A., Kamhawi, S., Voll, R., Klinger, M., Muller, A., Holscher, C., Herrmann, M., Sacks, D., Solbach, W. & Laskay, T. (2006) Leishmania disease development depends on the presence of apoptotic promastigotes in the virulent inoculum. *Proc Natl Acad Sci U S A*, 103, 13837-42.

Wang, Y. & Gu, X. (2001) Functional divergence in the caspase gene family and altered functional constraints: statistical analysis and prediction. *Genetics*, 158, 1311-20.

Wargo, A.R., Huijben, S., de Roode, J.C., Shepherd, J. & Read, A.F. (2007) Competitive release and facilitation of drug-resistant parasites after therapeutic chemotherapy in a rodent malaria model. *Proc Natl Acad Sci U S A*, 104, 19914-9.

Wessler, S.A., Diggle, S.P., Buckling, A., Gardner, A. & Griffin, A.S. (2007) The social lives of microbes. *Annu Rev Ecol Evol Syst*, 38, 53-77.

Wilson, D.S. (1975) A theory of group selection. *Proc Natl Acad Sci U S A*, 72, 143-6.

Yang, Z. (1997) PAML: a program package for phylogenetic analysis by maximum likelihood. *Comput Appl Biosci*, 13, 555-6.

Yang, Z. (2006) *Computational molecular evolution*. Oxford University Press, ISBN-13: 9780198567028 New York.

Yang, Z. (2007) PAML 4: phylogenetic analysis by maximum likelihood. *Mol Biol Evol*, 24, 1586-91.

Yang, Z. & Nielsen, R. (2000) Estimating synonymous and nonsynonymous substitution rates under realistic evolutionary models. *Mol Biol Evol*, 17, 32-43.

2

Drug Discovery into the 21ˢᵗ Century

Klaus Pors

Institute of Cancer Therapeutics, University of Bradford
UK

1. Introduction

Medicines discovery has come a long way since our ancient ancestors from the Neanderthals to the people of Mesopotamia, Egypt, Greece and China used herbal remedies to treat the sick people. In mediaeval times the quest for the *elixir of life* was pursued by alchemists, but it is the scientists of the past 100-150 years who have had success by translating laboratory-based discoveries into drugs that have literally saved countless millions of lives (Sneader, 2005). The German stock market collapsed in 1873 and it was during the recovery period that the upsurge in the economy lead to an expansion of chemical and electrical industries. The significant investment in the manufacture of synthetic dyes soon put Germany well ahead of all its competitors. As a consequence, German chemists did not only become very influential in the field of organic chemistry, but also led to the rise of the German pharmaceutical industry. Central to this industry were leading manufacturers including F. Bayer & Company and Farbenfabriken Hoechst who realised that their chemists researching and developing dyes also had the potential to produce new medicines (Sneader, 2005). One such scientist was Paul Ehrlich. Ehrlich was fascinated by colourful dyes and their capacity to interact with histological and cellular structures. Over several decades, he benefitted from chemical companies who provided hundreds to thousands of new dyes for his research. Given these dyes were biologically evaluated individually, the number of compounds probably exceeded the thousands or even millions of compounds being evaluated as a part of high-throughput screening (HTS) employed in academia and industry today. Ehrlich taught us that, in the broadest sense, the biological effect of a chemical compound such as a dye depends on its chemical composition and the cell on which it acts. He was able to establish a connection between chemistry, biology and medicine in an ingenious fashion; chemical dyes were the catalyst for this *revolutionary association* (Strebhardt & Ullrich, 2008). Simultaneous to his fascination of dyes, he also was inspired by his contemporaries carrying out research in immunology including Louis Pasteur, Robert Koch, Emil von Behring and Shibasaburo Kitasato. At the turn of the 20ᵗʰ century Ehrlich developed the receptor theory, which became instrumental to the understanding of how the binding of drugs to various types of receptors could occur due to structural differences in chemical compositions. He notably stated "Wir müssen chemisch zielen lernen" which translated to English equates "we have to learn how to aim chemically". Ehrlich's experiences with the treatment of infectious diseases with drugs derived from the German dye industry impelled him to look for ways of using organic chemistry to modify certain starting dyes in various ways to create new chemical structures with potential improved biological activity (Strebhardt & Ullrich, 2008). Erlich is often described as the founder of chemotherapy and his 'magic bullet concept' is still what today's scientists strive to aim for: to develop small molecules that attack pathogens yet remain harmless to healthy tissues.

During the two World Wars essential medicines normally supplied by Germany dried up and a gradual change in favour of synthetic drugs came about. Synthetic organic chemistry became an exceptional important discipline and is still one of the cornerstones of drug discovery. Synthetic organic chemistry has continually adapted to embrace innovative techniques and methodologies central to drug development. Much synthetic drug discovery emerged from cancer drug development and began with an observation that mustard gas, employed in chemical warfare during World Wars I and II, destroyed lymphatic tissue and bone marrow formation. The observations made by Drs. Gilman, Goodman and co-workers laid the foundation for conducting the first clinical trials with nitrogen mustards (β-chloroethylamines) in 1942 at Yale-New Haven Hospital, but a report of the clinical results was only made public four years later, due to the cloak of secrecy during World War II (Goodman et al, 1946; Hirsch, 2006). An array of DNA alkylating agents ensued, which paralleled an increased understanding of DNA in the 1950s. A number of other agents subsequently emerged, such as the vinca alkaloids and purine/pyrimidine synthesis inhibitors (Denny, 2002). These advances were, to a large extent, driven by the National Cancer Institute (NCI), enabling the assessment of primarily cytotoxic agents. By the 1970s, the importance of natural product-based early drug discovery had been realised (Denny, 2002). Unfortunately, the synthesis of many of these frequently promising, novel agents was often too complex and too expensive to allow progression into early stage clinical trials. This situation facilitated a paradigm shift whereby natural product screening was implemented into stage discovery initiatives, providing an opportunity to identify natural products as *bona fide* lead compounds. These leads were then subsequently developed into truncated molecules, which were more amenable to synthesis. More recently, advances in organic chemistry have successfully enabled the complete synthesis of many complex natural products, a milestone that has dramatically improved the ease with which chemists can now deal with the complexity of many of these naturally-derived architectural structures. Synthetic chemistry has also been instrumental in the development of drug delivery and prodrug strategies, which have focused on the development of selective therapeutics with reduced side-effect profiles (Brown & Wilson, 2004; Rooseboom et al, 2004). Although research in cancer medicines was the driver of much synthetic drug discovery it did run parallel with research against other diseases as illustrated in Figure 1.

Today, the emergence of the genomics era and the focus of events at the molecular level is changing the landscape of drug discovery. A wealth of convergent data that has caused many to not only speculate on an expanding druggable genome, but also given an optimism for grasping new opportunities to take drug discovery to the next level has become available (Billingsley, 2008). The number of gene products that are targets for existing drugs has been a topic for much debate and depends on the analysis performed, however, a valid estimate is in the region of 300-500 gene products (Overington et al, 2006). As the human genome is estimated to encode 20,000-25,000 human gene products, the number of drug targets is likely to increase. However, it will take some time to validate targets at the protein level, which has an added level of complexity. Both gene and protein expression profiling methodologies have been emerging over the last decade or so to monitor and catalogue changes in the expression of genes and their respective protein products. As such there are serious challenges ahead. Our understanding of human disease at the molecular level to elucidate changes in biochemical processes associated with disease phenotypes is of high significance. From a drug discovery point of view, the ultimate goal is to generate identifiable therapeutic targets while reducing drug development attrition.

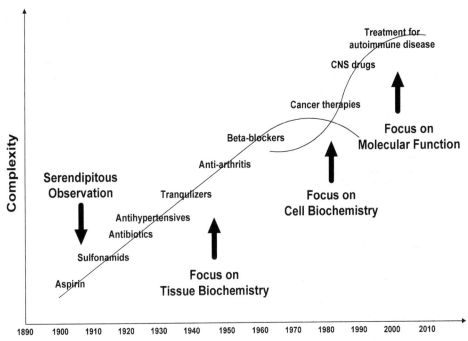

Fig. 1. Chronology of drug innovation. (Reprinted with permission from the Biopharmaceutical Industry Contributions to State and US Economics, available at www.milkeninstitute.org/pdf/biopharma_report.pdf, Milken Institute).

The mapping of the human genome was a gigantic landmark. Can scientists working at the interface of chemistry and biology in drug discovery utilise the data available to them to discover new ground-breaking drugs? Will the ever increasing cost of drug discovery halt the progression, especially in times of recession? Will research and development (R&D) in the emerging markets be an opportunity to climb to the next level of understanding in how to develop successful drugs? These are some of the questions that will be discussed in the following sections.

2. The evolution of modern drug discovery

At the beginning of the 20ᵗʰ century drug discovery was largely carried out by individuals such as Paul Ehrlich and his associates. This is now impossible, and requires teamwork encompassing members from various disciplines including chemistry, computational modelling, structural biology and pharmacology. This section outlines a general approach to drug discovery which has been dominant over the past couple of decades. The approach to drug design depends on the objectives of the design and investigational team, but will also depend to some extent on the disease that is targeted. The information available from the literature about a specific disease or target is used by the research team to decide what intervention would be most likely to bring about the desired result. The exact nature of the project progression depends on the resources available: for example, an academic group may not be as expansive as a large pharmaceutical company in terms of how to tackle the problems of validating a novel target or developing 'hit' and 'lead' compounds that will be able to modulate that target. The drug discovery process outlined in Figure 2 is, therefore, an approximate model which is employed by pharmaceutical companies, but one which a small biotech company or a university also can engage in through multiple collaborations. This discovery process can be instigated at several points and adapted to bring about the results needed to take a project to the next level. For a recent in-depth review of the early drug discovery process, see (Philpott *et al*, 2011).

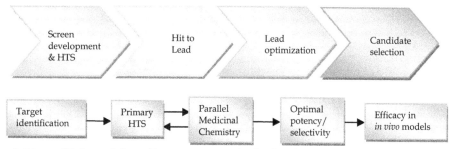

Fig. 2. The multi-faceted drug discovery process in the 21st Century.

Up until the mid 80s, drug discovery was focussed on isolation of natural products and medicinal chemistry was central for a research team to find more potent and selective compounds than the natural product or synthetic compound themselves. After isolation and characterisation of the natural products, structure-activity relationship (SAR) studies were and still are a vital tool in optimising a pharmacophore. Initially, a drug design process was an iterative course of action between the synthesis of new compounds by a synthetic/medicinal chemist and the screening of these for biological activity by a pharmacologist. The drug discovery process was chemistry-focussed rather than target-driven. As outlined in Figure 2, the discovery process of a drug now involves a multidisciplinary effort that is synergistic, which often encompasses HTS procedures. It is also one that often follows rules that are based on empirical findings from clinical investigations such as Lipinski's rule of 5 (Lipinski *et al*, 1997). 'Hit' compounds are progressed into a 'lead' compound, which undergoes thorough pharmacological and toxicological testing. The results of these tests enable a research team to decide whether it is profitable to continue with the progression of a specific project. The scenario is often to screen virtual or commercial libraries of compounds to identify hit molecules. The second stage is to prepare libraries of small molecules based around the hit molecule, measure their activity and correlate the results to determine the chemical structure with optimum activity. This analysis may make use of SARs, computational chemistry, combinatorial chemistry and enzymatic and cellular assays to help unravel biological activity derived from unique mechanism of action of a small molecule. The selection of a lead compound and the development of a synthetic pathway for its preparation on a large scale for preclinical and clinical investigations must also be considered at an early stage in the discovery process. If the lead molecule cannot be synthesised on a large scale progression to clinical evaluation will not be possible. Similarly, researchers must also devise suitable *in vitro* and *in vivo* tests to assess the activity and toxicity of the compounds produced. If there is no suitable way of testing a hit or lead molecule *in vivo* the project may come to a halt unless it is decided to spend resources on developing appropriate models.

Nowadays, hit and lead molecules with proven activity are assessed for susceptibility for phase I and II metabolism in the very early stages of the discovery process. For example, many HTS technologies are now available to detect cytochrome P450 (CYP) substrates or inhibitors, which should decrease the number of withdrawals of novel drugs from the market due to affinity for major CYP metabolising isozymes. HTS CYP data can be used to guide medicinal chemistry away from these interactions at an early stage and in certain cases might entirely solve the issue by targeted modification of the CYP interacting functionality (Zlokarnik *et al*, 2005).

HTS methodologies have been developed and have enabled research teams to generate vast numbers of compound variations of a desired pharmacophore. Combinatorial chemistry (combichem) was first applied to the generation of peptide arrays in 1984 and evolved rapidly into a new discipline that was hailed to revolutionise drug discovery (Lam & Renil, 2002). The early generations of combichem scientists captured the fascination of the industry, and coined or modified the common use of a number of buzzwords, phrases, and abbreviations that became widespread in the literature including deconvolution, diversomer, split-and-mix, multipin, SPOC or SPOS (solid-phase organic chemistry or synthesis), submonomer synthesis, T-bag (Teflon bag) to name a few (Moos *et al*, 2009). Interestingly, from the discovery point of view, the scientists working in the combichem environment require different management solutions to classical synthetic chemists. For example, chemists planning a traditional synthesis to obtain a target compound or a natural product typically conduct a retrosynthetic analysis to determine the best, and perhaps cheapest, way to obtain the target. In contrast, combinatorial chemists will primarily consider forward synthesis strategies that are founded in which building blocks are commercially available or indeed worth synthesising. Accordingly, chemical information systems that can be quickly accessed via updated databases of inventory and commercially available reagents are invaluable tools in reagent acquisition by the combinatorial chemists. While combichem matured from solid-phase synthesis to solid-supported synthesis, new synthetic strategies and techniques evolved. Some of these are now well integrated into the drug design process including microwave synthesis (Gedye *et al*, 1986), fluorous synthesis (Studer *et al*, 1997), click chemistry (Sharpless *et al*, 2001) and flow reactors (SalimiMoosavi *et al*, 1997). As with traditional drug design, combichem relies on organic synthesis methodologies and exploits automation and miniaturization to synthesize large libraries of compounds, which can accelerate the drug discovery process. The combinatorial approach is often systematic and repetitive, using sets of commercially available chemical reagents to form a diverse set of molecular entities. It is very powerful in early stage discovery and allows HTS to take place, combining rapid synthesis of chemical compounds to be screened using both enzymatic and cellular assays for evaluation. The quick turnaround of data allows a flow of information, which enables second and third generation of compounds to be generated in rapid fashion. Combichem mostly concerns "parallel" synthesis and "split-and-mix" synthesis (Figure 3).

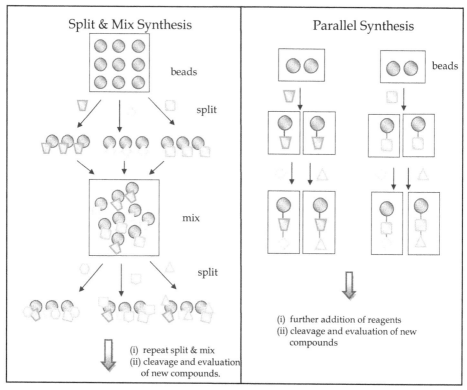

Fig. 3. Combinatorial chemistry approaches. The parallel synthesis is generally used to generate larger quantities of a small number of compounds and split and mix to generate smaller quantities of a larger number of molecules.

There is no doubt that combichem has become a mainstay tool of the drug discovery process. The strength of combinatorial techniques is based on the creation of large populations of molecules, or libraries that can be screened efficiently *en masse* in a short period of time. The vast amounts of money spent on development of combinatorial techniques have not yet resulted in many drug successes. The only real success story at present is the development of the multikinase inhibitor sorafenib, which now has been approved for clinical use by the *Food and Drug Administration (FDA)* for the treatment of advanced renal cancer (Wilhelm *et al*, 2006). However, combichem has spun out many exciting technologies that now occupy a central place in the biotech industry. The mapping of the human genome may have provided a new area of application of combichem in combination with other HTS methodologies including techniques and instruments developed for DNA microarrays. Indeed, high-density chemical microarrays can now be synthesized *in situ* on glass slides or be printed through covalent linkage or non-specific adsorption to the surface of the solid-support with fully automatic arrays. In conjunction with the one-bead one-compound combinatorial library method, chemical microarrays have proven to be very valuable in 'hit' identification and 'lead' optimization. HTS protein expression systems, robust high-density protein, peptide and small-molecule microarray systems, and automatic mass spectrometers are essential tools for the field of functional proteomics (Lam & Renil, 2002). In despite of this more focussed approach to drug discovery, combichem has been disappointing in delivering drugs to the market (Rydzewski, 2008). One of the main reasons is that combichem has been built on peptide chemistry that now has use in protein and nucleotide research, but which is not best suited to producing orally active drugs (Moos *et al.*, 2009). Another limitation of combichem is that small molecules developed via this technique do not cover broad *chemical space*. When comparing the properties of compounds in combichem libraries to those of approved drugs and natural products, it has been observed that combichem libraries suffer particularly from the lack of chirality, as well as structure rigidity, both of which are widely regarded as drug-like properties (Feher & Schmidt, 2003). Since the enormous success with natural products as drugs or use for drug development in the 70-80s, it has not been fashionable by the pharmaceutical industry to use these as leads for drug development. Often because of the complex structural architecture of natural products, which make them difficult to synthesise in the laboratory on a large scale basis. However, what cannot be disputed is that natural products cover much chemical diversity. As chirality and rigidity are the two most important features distinguishing approved drugs and natural products from compounds in combichem libraries, these are the two issues that are essential components of diversity-oriented synthesis (DOS) that aim at coverage of the chemical space, instead of libraries consisting of colossal numbers of compounds.

2.1 Discovery of small molecules to explore biological pathways and uncover new targets

The mapping of the human genome, the improved understanding of both pathological causes and function of biological targets and the development of HTS technologies ought to have resulted in a higher number of new chemical entities (NMEs) for medicinal use. So why has this not been the case? There may be several reasons, which will now be considered. Computational molecular modelling has provided scientists with an insight into biochemical events at the molecular level. An understanding of the binding process of small molecules to many macromolecules such as DNA is well understood, however the same cannot be said about other targets. Many stones are still left unturned, perhaps due to the lack of interest or belief that so-called "undruggable" proteins can be successfully targeted. It has been estimated that only 10-14% of the proteins encoded in the human genome are 'druggable' using existing 'drug-like' molecules (Hopkins & Groom, 2002). However, given that the *chemical space*, the complete set of all possible small molecules, has been calculated to comprise 10^{30}–10^{200} structures depending on the parameters used (Bauer *et al*, 2010) there are an incredible number of yet uncovered chemical structures. Considering the limitations of chemical libraries in addressing challenging targets, it is important to recognize that the vast majority of accessible libraries of small molecules are based on existing drugs (Moura-Letts *et al*, 2011). Drugging targets that are within our capacity to accept as targets and exercising principles such as Lipinski's "rule of five" that have yielded success in the past is safe territory, so it is perfectly understandable that we want to continue such lines of research. "Me too" compounds are likely to give pharmaceutical companies a financial return and academic scientists may obtain grant funding if the proposed research makes sense. Grant reviewers can appreciate the hypotheses and the scientific methodologies and may be inclined to fund projects that will give an outcome of sorts. However, it also appears that industry, research councils and other funding bodies want to keep an element of blue-sky research – they just don't want to fund it. Historically we know that serendipity has played a major part of most success stories. So to cut out funding that is not to support blue-sky but mainstream research is likely to have profound consequences. Although Lipinski's "rule of five" has merit and a place in drug discovery it may also be an Achilles heel in progressing new drug discovery projects (Abad-Zapatero, 2007). Why? A drawback is that the shape and size of drugs become limited. Unless carefully used, HTS technologies such as combichem will continue to only generate low hit rates, particularly when screening against challenging targets (Boehringer et al, 2000; Edwards et al, 2007). Additionally, optimisation of lead compounds can be problematic owing to the often large and relatively lipophilic nature of the screening hits (Chessari & Woodhead, 2009a). Wise men will always use experiences from the past and present, but discovery of NMEs must also entail trespassing new horizons or in the drug discovery world, new chemical space.

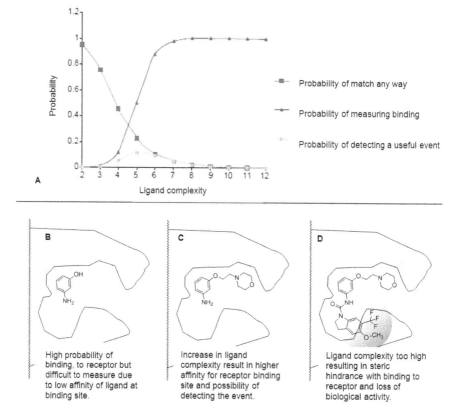

Fig. 4. (A) Success landscape for a binding site of ligands with increasing molecular complexity. (Reprinted with permission from Zartler & Shapiro, *Curr. Opin. Chem. Biol.* 2005, 9(4), 366-370, copyright (2005) Elsevier and *J.Chem. Inf. Comput. Sci.* 2001, 41, 856-864, copyright (2001), American Chemical Society). (B-D) An example of increase in ligand complexity using 3-aminophenol as starting material.

An insight into the difficulties in successful drug development is provided by Hann and co-workers who in their study suggest that if a drug discovery process starts with very simple chemical structures, then there is a better chance of finding both detectable binding and a unique binding mode. Similarly, lead molecules that are simpler also give more available chemical space for optimization, especially in light of the properties that are needed for oral bioavailability (Zartler & Shapiro, 2005). Figure 4A shows the trade off between detecting binding and a unique match. Essentially, the chance of finding a detectable and unique binding mode is dependent on the chance of determining binding and the chance of having a distinctive binding mode or match. For example, if 3-aminphenol was a ligand in a screening collection, there would be a high probability of it binding, but due to low affinity and time of occupancy at the binding site, it would be difficult to detect any such binding (Figure 4B). If 3-aminophenol was further reacted to afford 3-(2-morpholinoethoxy)aniline, the complexity of this ligand would increase and the probability of the binding would increase as a result. However, if the aniline amine moiety was derivatised with a fluorinated indoline to generate a ligand of high complexity, steric hindrance would hamper any binding in this specific receptor model (Figure 4D). By increasing the molecular complexity of a ligand the chance of measuring the binding is enhanced, but at the same time such modifications may also augment the likelihood of negative interactions (Zartler & Shapiro, 2005).

One approach toward broadening our understanding of the relationship between structure and function of a target protein is to generate many new small molecules, simple in shape and size, which are in accordance with Hann's study, that modulate the proteins' functions. This enables the study of the interactions of ligand and protein. The past 10 years have seen the screening of specific components of small molecules evolve from a niche area of research to become an important tool known as fragment-based drug discovery (FBDD). Fragments are defined as low molecular weight (MW <300), moderately lipophilic (clogP < 3) and highly soluble organic molecules (Chessari & Woodhead, 2009a). As a consequence, medicinal chemists use hit compounds to probe new chemical space in a number of ways as illustrated in Figure 5.

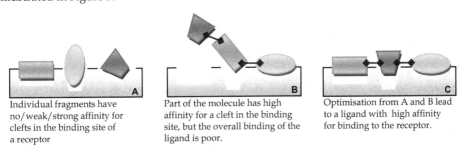

| Individual fragments have no/weak/strong affinity for clefts in the binding site of a receptor | Part of the molecule has high affinity for a cleft in the binding site, but the overall binding of the ligand is poor. | Optimisation from A and B lead to a ligand with high affinity for binding to the receptor. |

Fig. 5. Fragment-based drug discovery.

The first medicinal chemistry approaches employing FBDD as a key component of the discovery process can be traced back 15-20 years. In contrast to combichem, FBDD strategies have had a more rapid impact in terms of developing drugs with clinical potential. The wide variety of contexts in which FBDD is now being used (SAR-by-NMR, HTX, scaffold-hopping, selectivity mapping) illustrates its practical utility in mainstream medicinal chemistry. The promise of more resourceful technology has fuelled enthusiasm for FBDD, which is design intensive and enabled by structural biology. Indeed, screening fragments, particularly when using sensitive biophysical techniques may also allow scientists to tackle some of the more challenging drug discovery targets. Fragment libraries statistically cover chemical space better than drug-like or lead-like libraries and as a consequence fewer compounds need to be screened. Also fragment-based screening tends to deliver high hit rates with the additional benefit of providing multiple start points for optimisation programmes (Chessari & Woodhead, 2009a).

FBDD's recent successes outlined in Table 1 (Chessari & Woodhead, 2009b) indicate that use of this design intensive drug discovery approach is delivering results that have paved the way to clinical evaluation and it may not be long before the first drug reaches the marketplace (de Kloe *et al*, 2009).

Compound	Company	Target	Progress	Detection method
ABT-263	Abbott	Bcl-X_L	Phase 2	NMR
AT9283	Astex	Aurora	Phase 2	X-ray
LY-517717	Lilly/Protherics	FXa	Phase 2	Computation/X-ray
NVP-AUY-922	Novartis/Vernalis	Hsp90	Phase 2	NMR
Indeglitazar	Plexxikon	PPAR antagonist	Phase 2	HCS/X-ray
ABT-518	Abbott	MMP-2 & 9	Phase 1	NMR
AT7519	Astex	CDK2	Phase 1	X-ray
AT13387	Astex	Hsp90	Phase 1	NMR/X-ray
IC-776	Lilly/ICOS	LFA-1	Phase 1	NMR
PLX-4032	Plexxikon	B-RafV[600E]	Phase 1	HCS/X-ray
PLX-5568	Plexxikon	Kinase Inhibitor	Phase 1	HCS/X-ray
SGX-523	SGX Pharmaceuticals	Met	Phase 1	X-ray/HCS
SNS-314	Sunesis	Aurora	Phase 1	MS

Table 1. Fragment derived compounds and furthest stage of clinical development.
(Adapted with permission from Chessari & Woodhead, From fragment to clinical candidate-a historical perspective. *Drug Discov Today*, 2009, 14(13-14), 668-675, copyright (2009) Elsevier).

2.2 Exploring chemical space

Drug discovery today critically depends on HTS of compound libraries *in silico* and *in vitro*. Novel chemical structures (also known as chemotypes) are of particular interest since these might display different properties to drug-like small molecules and may be used to interrogate biological pathways. Unfortunately, most approaches to create new compounds rely on using commercially-available known starting materials or building blocks and utilise existing reactions to generate small molecules, which are not well-suited to uncover novel chemotypes (Reymond & Fink, 2007). A change to the discovery of small molecules that possess biological activity, but are under-represented in commercial screening collections may provide suitable fragments for further development. An analysis by Stoichet and co-workers (Shoichet *et al*, 2009) revealed amongst other things that currently commercially-available compounds and libraries have more in common with compounds derived from natural products and metabolites than with a virtual library of 26.4 million molecules (chemotypes containing of up to 11 atoms of C, N, O, and F comprising 110.9 million stereoisomers). Is this a surprise? Stoichet argued that the reason current libraries are effective at all in identifying new chemotypes is that they are based, albeit largely unintentionally, on structures in naturally occurring molecules, which have coevolved with proteins that bind them.

In a recent study, Tan and co-workers analysed 40 top-selling small molecule drugs (39 of which are orally bioavailable), a collection of 60 diverse natural products (including the 24 identified by Ganesan as having led to an approved drug from 1970 to 2006) and 20 drug-like compounds from ChemBridge and ChemDiv. Each compound was analyzed for 20 calculated structural and physicochemical parameters, and then principal component analysis was used to replot the data in a 2-dimensional format representing 73% of the information in the full 20-dimensional dataset (for full details, see (Bauer *et al*, 2010).

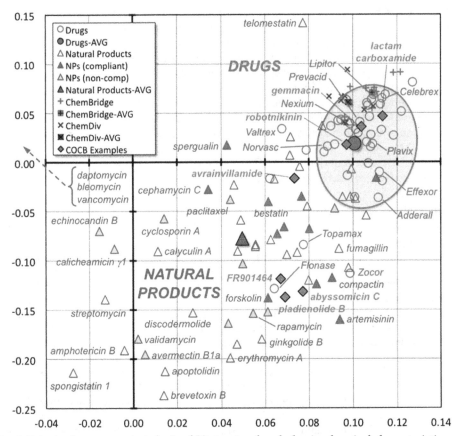

Fig. 6. Principal component analysis of 20 structural and physicochemical characteristics of 40 top-selling drugs (red circles), 60 natural products (blue triangles), including Ganesan's rule-of-five compliant (pink filled) and non-compliant (blue filled) subsets, and 20 compounds from commercial drug-like libraries (ChemBridge, pink plusses; Chem Div, maroon crosses). The two unitless, orthogonal axes represent 73% of the information in the full 20-dimensional dataset. Recent examples of natural products and library-derived probes that address challenging targets discussed herein are also shown (green diamonds). (Reprinted with permission from Bauer *et. al.*, Expanding the range of 'druggable' targets with natural product-based libraries: an academic perspective. *Curr. Opin. Chem. Biol.*, 2010, 14(3), 308-314, copyright (2009) Elsevier).

Putting the details aside, the key message from this data representation (Figure 6) is that the top-selling drugs are located as a cluster in a specific area of the plot with the drug-like libraries overlapping the same regional zone. Moreover, the few outlier drugs are natural products or derivatives, and these molecules, along with the 60 natural products, span a much broader range of chemical space. In part, this study points to natural products as chemical architectures that not only cover chemical space best but also are likely to be suitable for developing probe and drug-like molecules that can modulate macromolecular proteins in various ways.

Small molecules have great potential to aid the process of understanding and improving human health. Accordingly, there is much incentive for using small molecules to explore new chemical space by employing methodologies that are aimed at exploring unchartered waters and leaving well-researched areas behind, but by no means forgotten. As we have seen, FBDD is beginning to prove that developing technologies outside mainstream medicinal chemistry can be fruitful. Aware of the fact that bioactivity is not randomly dispersed in the vast chemical space, chemists have been cultivating hypotheses that can bring them closer to the islands of bioactivities. Natural products have always been a source of inspiration and their structural motifs provide biologically relevant starting points for library synthesis to generate new molecules integrating pharmacophores known to produce biological activity. In addition to FBDD, emerging tools to guide compound discovery include diversity-oriented synthesis and chemical genetics.

2.2.1 Diversity-oriented synthesis

Diversity-oriented synthesis (DOS) aims to synthesize small molecules that cover incongruent targets in a multidimensional descriptor space (Burke & Schreiber, 2004). Essentially what this means is that multiple regions in a confined chemical space are targeted with small molecules often comprising a fragment of a pharmacophore with proven biological activity. Such collections are also essential to chemical genetics, which is discussed further below (section 2.1.2.). DOS is built on a solid platform comprising traditional medicinal chemistry but can also incorporate HTS technologies such as combichem. Essentially, drug discovery of small molecules can be categorized into three approaches that cover chemical space differently: The first approach uses target-oriented synthesis (TOS) and resembles a well-trodden path that relies primarily on nature to discover molecules with useful, macromolecule-perturbing properties. After isolation and characterisation, natural products possessing biological activity become a target for chemical synthesis. Using conventional synthetic chemistry based on retrosynthetic planning, the aim of TOS is to populate a discrete point in chemical space that is known to yield biological activity (Figure 7A). The second approach uses either medicinal chemistry or combichem and aims to explore chemistry space that is in close vicinity to a precise region known to have useful properties (Figure 7B). The source of the starting or lead compounds can vary and may include a natural product, a known drug or pharmacophore, or a rationally designed structure derived from i.e. a crystal structure of a macromolecule of interest. The aim in this approach is to access diversity to some degree using diverse building blocks and usually involves synthesising analogues of a given target structure using retrosynthetic planning. The synthesis effort in DOS aims to create a broad distribution of compounds in chemistry space (Figure 7C), including currently poorly populated (or even vacuous) space, and in the future, space found empirically to correlate best with desired properties. Synthesis pathways employed in DOS are branched and divergent, and they are planned in the forward-synthetic direction (Bender *et al*, 2006; Burke & Schreiber, 2004; Spring *et al*, 2008).

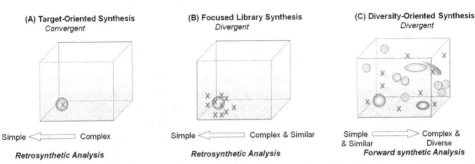

Fig. 7. TOS, focused library synthesis and DOS; a comparison of the planning strategies used (i.e. retrosynthetic or forward synthetic analysis and convergent or divergent synthesis) and the chemical space interrogated (i.e. focused point/area or diverse coverage). (Adapted with permission from Spring *et. al.* (2008) Diversity-oriented synthesis; a spectrum of approaches and results. *Organic & Biomolecular Chemistry*, 2008, 6(7), 1149-1158. Available at http://dx.doi.org/10.1039/B719372F, Copyright, The Royal Society of Chemistry (2008).

As described in two prominent reviews (Burke & Schreiber, 2004; Spring *et al*, 2008), skeletal diversity can be achieved principally in two ways. The first method involves the use of different reagents and a common building block as starting point. This 'reagent-based approach' is also known as a branching pathway. The second method or the 'substrate-based approach' uses different building blocks that contain pre-encoded information of desired architectural geometry which are subjected to a common set of conditions leading to a diverse set of small molecules (Figure 8). Although there are not many successes at this point in time, DOS is used increasingly as an attempt to probe biological pathways or develop NMEs. Conceptually, it is important to appreciate that it is the functional diversity and not the structural diversity of small molecules that is a key measure of success in the application of DOS. For specific chemical strategies of DOS application, see for example (Burke & Schreiber, 2004; Hanson *et al*, 2010; Nielsen & Schreiber, 2008b; Spandl *et al*, 2008).

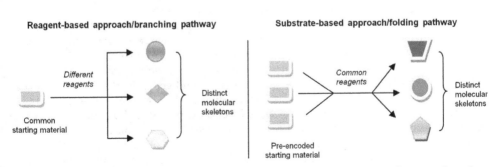

Fig. 8. Two common approaches for achieving skeletal diversity in DOS is "reagent-based approach/branching pathway" and "substrate-based approach/folding pathway".

2.2.2 Chemical genetics

In many ways, modern genetics began with the applied and theoretical work of the nature of inheritance in plants by German-Czech scientist Gregor Mendel in the mid-19th century. In comparison, the science in chemical genetics is only a couple of decades old, but has been gaining momentum in recent years. Chemical genetics has very much its origin in classical genetics and uses most of the methods and terminology already established. Genetic knockouts have been key to illustrating biological pathways and causations of pathological diseases and now the fields of chemical biology and related modern fields are enabling small molecules to be discovered and developed and used as chemical 'knockdowns'. To understand a system, you need to perturb it. This principle underlies most of the experimental sciences and explains why our depth of understanding of biological systems has been largely determined by the availability of tools that can be used to disrupt them (Stockwell, 2004). In order to close the genotype-phenotype gap, biological research has to reach beyond genomics, proteomics, and dissection of biological systems into their prime constituents (Bon & Waldmann, 2010). Protein function is regulated in complex networks with other biomacromolecules, small molecules and supramolecular structures like membranes (Zamir & Bastiaens, 2008). Whereas genetic manipulation results in a permanent alteration of the native structure of the network, chemical perturbations with small molecule modulators of protein function provides temporal control using dose-response explorations without fundamentally transforming the biological network (Stockwell, 2004). It is very attractive to use small molecules to perturb a biological system because of their dynamic nature, which offers many advantages: (i) ability to target a single domain of a multidomain protein, (ii) allows precise temporal control that is critical for rapidly acting processes, (iii) can target orthologous or paralogous proteins, enabling comparisons between species or redundant functions, and (iv) do not directly alter the concentrations of a targeted protein, thus avoiding indirect effects on multiprotein complexes (Lehar *et al*, 2008a).

The small molecules used to probe biological networks are ideally developed by mainstream medicinal chemistry and increasingly supported by modern methodologies such as DOS in order to encompass regions of chemical space that are not defined by existing screening collections as discussed previously. Essentially, chemical genetic studies can be designed to be either *forward* or *reverse* depending on the direction of learning that underlies their motivation (Nghiem & Kawasumi, 2007; Stockwell, 2004). *Forward* studies involve evaluating many chemical probes against one or a few phenotypes in order to identify active compounds, and reverse studies execute multiple phenotype measurements on a few related chemical probes to characterize their function. In both cases, the chemical probes can be analyzed across a panel of phenotypic assays to identify either broad activity or selectivity between the phenotypes (Lehar *et al*, 2008a). To elevate the complexity of the test system to reflect for example upon a diseased state of a cell combination chemical genetics (CCG) can be employed. CCG can be defined as the systematic testing of multiple perturbations involving chemical probes and can include either chemical combinations or mixed chemical and genetic perturbations. Classical and chemical genetics (Figure 9) are generally divided into *forward* screens, in which uncharacterized perturbers are tested against a selected phenotype to detect genes associated with that phenotype, and *reverse* studies, in which a specific gene or protein is modulated and multiple phenotypes are monitored to determine the effects of that specific target (Nghiem & Kawasumi, 2007; Stockwell, 2004). Studies involving combined perturbations can be similarly classified with the mechanistic focus shifted from individual targets to interactions between them (Lehar *et al*, 2008b).

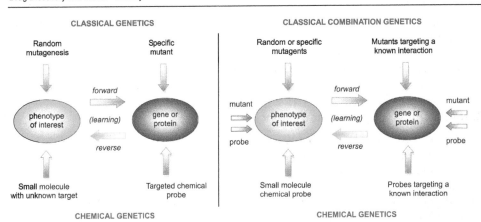

Fig. 9. Combined perturber studies in the context of forward and reverse genetics. The essence of classical and chemical genetics is to explore the function of individual genes or proteins. In combination chemical genetics, the focus of investigations shifts from individual targets to interactions between them or conditional target dependencies, and the perturbations are applied as combinations. (Adapted with permission from Lehar *et. al.* Combination chemical genetics. *Nat. Chem. Biol.* 2008, 4 (11), 674-681, copyright 2008, Macmillan Publishers Ltd).

Chemical biology has clearly made an impact in drug discovery and great strides towards offering new technologies that can progress our understanding of human health has been made. Given the temporal control offered by small molecules and the ability to use combinations of small molecule modulators, chemical genetics promises to complement the use of pure genetic analysis to study a wide range of biological systems. Chemical genetics aims to answer questions in complex test systems and may provide the field with commercial chemical probes that can be used to probe pathways and elucidate more about biological targets. The discovery of the potent and selective deacetylase inhibitors tubacin and histacin are examples of how powerful DOS and chemical genetics can be in combination with computational methods such as principal component analysis (Haggarty *et al*, 2003). However, good chemical probes for *in vitro* and especially *in vivo* perturbation are not easy to come by as small molecules are generally pleiotropic and they have multiple dose-dependent molecular targets that are often not fully characterized, which leads to unexpected activities. Obstacles and challenges are similar to those in drug development: small molecules often have inherent problems such as *in vitro* aggregation, poor solubility, difficulty in crossing biological membranes and reactive or toxic functionalities. At present, development of chemical probes for *in vivo* testing may be too ambitious a goal. As a result, evaluation of the effect of chemical 'knockdowns' in clinically relevant tissue should in the near future be in more complex assays that mimic for example malignant tissue. 3D cell culture technologies are increasingly becoming essential to *in vitro* screening. High content screening (HCS) has improved cell-based assays by combining high-resolution digital imaging with powerful software algorithms to increase the amount of data produced per well. 3D cell culture will not only empower HCS by supporting *in vivo* morphologies with current cell types, but also enable the use of primary and stem cells in drug discovery. Regardless of the challenges, primary and stem cells will become the focal point of 3D cell culture in the coming years (Justice *et al*, 2009), which could take chemical genetics to the next level. In summary the success of chemical genetics heavily relies on the availability of chemical libraries that offer structural diversity of small molecules that possess biological activity and complement libraries of compounds based on drugs and natural products (Lehar *et al*, 2008a). However, there is still a gap between developing commercial probes and inventing innovative drugs to treat illnesses.

3. R&D is moving global but will innovation increase?

"Trying to invent new drugs is no picnic." Sir James Black (1924-2010).
Only a small percentage of design and construction of scientific hypotheses that form the basis for a project actually yield exciting lead agents, let alone NMEs. Although the level of investment in pharmaceutical research and development (R&D) has increased dramatically since 1950 to US$50 billion per year at present, the number of new drugs that are approved annually is no greater now than it was in those days (Munos, 2009). From 1950 to 2008, the FDA approved 1,222 new drugs comprising of NMEs or new biologics (Figure 10). Historically, only approximately 1 out of 15–25 drug candidates survives the detailed safety and efficacy testing (in animals and humans) required for a drug to become a marketed product. As if these numbers were not disconcerting enough, from the industry's point of view, of the few drug candidates that successfully become marketed products, only one in three will become a major commercial product (Zhao & Guo, 2009). The discovery and development of a drug has often been quoted to take 10-15 years and cost in the region of $800 million to bring to market although the exact figure is probably much lower; i.e. the cost of NMEs is no doubt very high and close to $800 million but in contrast "me-too" drugs where most research has already been established the costs are nowhere near this figure (Angell, 2004). Regardless of the exact cost of developing a drug, the process of its development is a high-stakes, long-term and risky activity that has few peers in the commercial world, but the potential benefits to the millions of patients with serious diseases provide a constant motivating force for everybody involved in drug discovery.
A closer analysis reveals that 28 small-molecule first-in-class NMEs that entered the market between 1999 and 2008 were first discovered using phenotypic evaluation methods such as the employment of cell-based or whole-organism assays (Figure 11). Moreover, 17 NMEs were from target-based approaches and 5 NMEs were derived from natural substances. In contrast, 83 (51%) of the 164 follower drugs were discovered via target-based approaches. A possible contributing factor to this trend could have been a lag time between the introduction of new technologies and strategies, and their impact in terms of the number of approved first-in-class NMEs derived from such approaches. However, such a lag is not strongly apparent in a comparison of the cumulative number of NMEs from the two approaches during the period analysed (Swinney & Anthony, 2011).

3.1 Investment in education is vital to innovation
The investment in R&D has increased substantially in recent decades in efforts to obtain favourable market position and exclusivity in terms of IP position. The annual number of truly innovative new medicines approved by the FDA is not on the rise as highlighted in the previous section. Given the embracement of HTS technologies including combichem and FBDD combined with the improved understanding of disease pathogenesis, it is disappointing that there is no apparent evidence of an increase in the number of NMEs

approved. An immediate answer is related to the accelerating costs of R&D which hampers progression of many research projects. Another deep-rooted answer may be related to education policies: how pupils in schools as well as both under- and postgraduate students in universities are being taught in the chemical, physical & biological sciences. Firstly, the development of HTS is costly and therefore largely inaccessible to academia that often carries out drug discovery on a shoe-string budget. One consequence is that academia, who historically has been the driver of much innovation, will feel not only compelled to lower

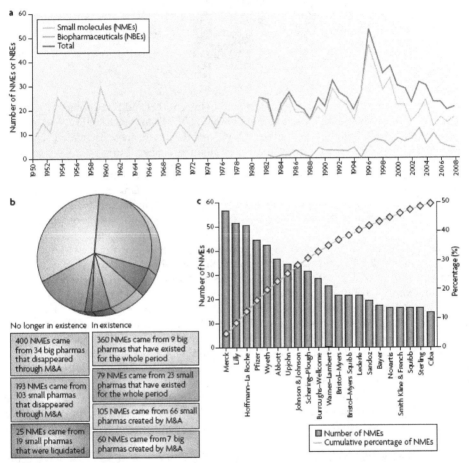

Fig. 10. Origins of new drugs. (a) Timeline of approvals of NMEs and new biological entities (NBEs) by the FDA between 1950 and 2008. (b) Characteristics of the 261 organizations that have produced the 1,222 NMEs approved since 1950. (c) 21 companies have produced half of all the NMEs that have been approved since 1950, although half of these companies no longer exist. In (b) and (c), both new small molecules and new biologics are grouped as NMEs for simplicity. M&A, mergers and acquisitions. (Reprinted with permission from Munos, B. Lessons from 60 years of pharmaceutical innovation. *Nature reviews.* 2009, 8 (12), 959-968, copyright 2009, Macmillan Publishers Ltd).

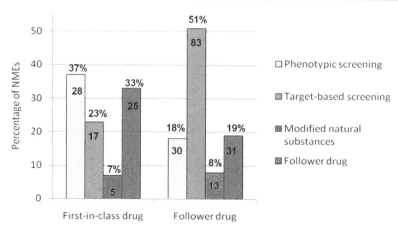

Fig. 11. The distribution of new drugs discovered between 1999 and 2008, according to the discovery strategy. The graph illustrates the number of NMEs in each category. (Adapted with permission from Swinney & Anthony. How were new medicines discovered? *Nature reviews*. 2011, 10(7), 507-519, copyright 2011, Macmillan Publishers Ltd).

their ambitions, but also hand over the baton to pharma- and biotech companies when it comes to innovative initiatives; that would be disastrous for many reasons. In particular, students would not be educated in using cutting-edge equipment and HTS technologies. Secondly, the approval of NMEs is also affected by the demonstration of adequate clinical safety and efficacy in humans which has become more complex, and ever-increasing amounts of data are now required by regulatory agencies (Lombardino & Lowe, 2004). Thirdly, it could also be argued that the dwindling supply of new drugs is related to a decrease in output by stifling the creativity of the scientists involved in drug discovery? This statement requires a more comprehensive discussion. In the western world the funding climate of academic institutions has changed and the pharmaceutical industry, in spite of scaling back on research operations and sizeable job cuts in 2010 (Mullin, 2010), is slowly returning to the funding levels available pre-recession and the international banking collapse in September 2008. For example, the UK funding landscape is having an impact on attracting and training students in synthetic organic chemistry. Many medicinal chemists working in the biotech and pharmaceutical industries received their PhDs in organic synthesis, a consequence of the view that excellence in organic synthesis is a prerequisite for a successful medicinal chemistry career (Frantz, 2003). However, the rise in small biotech companies has resulted in a demand for scientists that have research experience in multidisciplinary disciplines, and a broader education than in a single area such as synthetic organic chemistry (Pittman, 2010). Obtaining funding for chemical sciences may become more challenging in the future, due to a shift away from "responsive mode" applications; the success rate of EPSRC (the main British funding body for chemical sciences) applications has dropped from approx. 25% to 10% (Crow, 2008), and this coincided with a recent policy to limit applications from persistently unsuccessful academics (Lewcock, 2009). The EPSRC plans to cut research grant expenditure by £61 million to £372 million between 2010-2011 and 2014-2015. It will also stop accepting grant proposals regarding funding for PhD students by 2012, which instead will be supported exclusively through Centres for Doctoral Training Accounts (DTAs). Although, this shift provides a small £13 million rise in funding for studentships through to 2015 to offset the research grant decline it is potential very damaging for British universities that do not hold DTAs (Extance, 2011).

Restricting support is likely to result in a reduction of the pool of potential answers/solutions to critical problems, which arise from current and future challenges. This has led to concerns within industry that a reduced emphasis on organic synthesis would negatively impact the quality of future generations of scientists working at the interface of chemistry and biology (Pors *et al*, 2009). To balance these changes the EPSRC has initiated "grand challenges", where money is available to address key priorities for future collaborative research, such as in human health. These funding policy changes present opportunities for academics that can adapt, and a likely consequence is an increased degree of collaboration between organic synthesis and other disciplines. Ultimately this may result in the establishment of highly collaborative centres focused on chemical biology, drug discovery and other disciplines that support this important thematic initiative. One concern that industry has with such collaborative centres is that the students may find it more difficult to acquire highly specialised physical and synthetic organic chemistry skills and/or tools that would allow them to compete in a highly competitive job market. If, however, these centres do provide a thorough educational opportunity these PhD students may prove to be highly qualified for a career in medicinal chemistry and chemical biology, where success in projects frequently relies upon the successful collaboration and integration of multiple disciplines that are necessary for not only combating the major diseases, but also for becoming leaders in innovation (Pors *et al*, 2009).

Martin Schuurmann, the chairman of the European Institute of Innovation and Technology (EIT), has recently (Burke, 2011) opinionated that although Europe is a leader in research, it is not often in innovation. He believes that there are several reasons for this: a lack of education in entrepreneurship; too great a focus on research alone, rather than on the triangle' of education, research and business; a lack of focus on entrepreneurship as the key driver for innovation; and a weak leadership, typically embodied by committees. Although Schuurmann was talking broadly about innovation, there is no doubt that education and experience in entrepreneurship is vital to innovation in drug discovery too. Europe currently offers insufficient opportunities for young investigators to progress independent careers and to make the transition from assisting supervisors/projects leader to being independent researchers in their own right. As a consequence, highly talented research scientists are being hold back in their career progression and there is also a danger that these promising young scientists are encouraged to seek advancement outside the continent. In an attempt to maintain the best scientists of the future generations in Europe, the European Union has established *Starting Independent Researcher Grants* (ERC Starting Grants), which aim to support up-and-coming research leaders who are about to establish or consolidate a proper research team and to start conducting independent research in Europe. The budgets for the 2009 and 2010 calls were €325 and €580 million with a successful funding rate around 15% and 10% respectively for the two calls (European Research Council, 2011). The low success rate suggests high competition across Europe to obtain such prestigious grants, but is actually favourable to scientists working in *Life Sciences* where around 35% of the total funding was allocated in both 2009 and 2010. As such the European Union recognises the importance of research at the chemistry/biological interface, which in part underpins drug discovery.

While the system for funding students is slightly different in the USA, similar challenges and obstacles remain for principal investigators and the students in their laboratories. Take the example of cancer drug discovery, the National Cancer Institute, which is part of the National Institutes of Health (NIH) and the U.S. Department of Health and Human Services (DHHS), remains the principal agency for cancer research with other research grant support available from the Center for Disease Control (CDC) and Prevention and the Department of Defence (DOD) (National Cancer Institute, 2011a). The NCI is one of 27 Institutes and Centres that make up the NIH annual operating budget, which is allocated by the US Congress has remained flat at approximately $4.8 billion since 2004 (National Cancer Institute, 2011b); a number that has drastically lowered the funding payline with success rates for new Research Project Grants (better known as a RO1 grant) currently at or below 10% in year 2008 and 2009 (U.S. Department of Health & Human Services, 2010). While scientists earlier in their career are often supported for a period of 3-5 years through several financial mechanisms including foundations and academic departments, the current funding situation remains dichotomised given these significant federal budget constraints. While there is an appreciated need to support those in the earliest stage of their career the risk-reward equation from the viewpoint of many of these funding agencies is one that does not currently support innovative or highly translational research programs. Unfortunately, these programs are often the foundation of budding young scientists in drug discovery. With no or very little funding available to fund young academics there is a widespread concern in both the UK and US that innovative initiatives are stagnant or even on the decline. Indirectly, the tough financial times in Europe and the US may benefit the emerging countries such as China. Because of its traditional education philosophy and the "one-child" policy of the past 30 years, Chinese parents are eager to educate their child in the best possible institutions and invest between RMB 10,000-15,000 (USD 1,200-1,800) per year of study in higher education (Lian, 2005). This is a substantial amount of money that a lot of families have to borrow, but ensures a hard-working mentality and ability to survive that benefit project leaders in governmental and industrial research environments. These qualities coupled with a desire to learn from the West are central to education of the newer generations of students in China and ultimately to the establishment of the Pharma industry and rapid increase in the numbers of smaller biotech companies.

Whether in Europe, the US or in the emerging countries, new strategies are emerging as a result of re-focusing and restructuring of the drug discovery field, leading to a new 'front end' between pharma and academia which aims at more successfully taking new therapeutic entities through pre-clinical and clinical development to the market (Tralau-Stewart et al, 2009). By addressing "grand challenges" such as in healthcare and in setting up collaborative centres with a focus on drug discovery it may be that academia can benefit from advice and support from the pharmaceutical and biotech industries given their longstanding success in this field. During difficult economic times, however, many private sector companies are forced to reduce their R&D budgets. This is an opportunity for academics to fill an important innovation gap. In the business sector we are witnessing this change through the significant licensing as well as merger and acquisition activity that has been documented through numerous partnership deals between academic institutions and pharmaceutical companies. The goals of academia and industry may become more closely aligned if, as suggested by the research councils of the UK, there is a shift in academia from fundamental/basic research towards knowledge transfer and innovation. The EPSRC, for instance, encourages the formation of partnerships between academia and industry through its postgraduate CASE awards, which already serve to strengthen the ties between the two. Industry also contributes in a positive manner to undergraduate teaching of medicinal chemistry in many universities through educational tools, including industrial case histories as well as more traditional academic lecturers. However, some people in industry have the opinion that many of the key skills and novel techniques that are a part of modern drug discovery in industry are lacking at undergraduate level (Frantz, 2003). The challenge for universities is to ensure that the medicinal chemistry content of their chemistry courses is relevant to modern drug discovery and to address the opportunity for greater collaboration between industry and academia. Given the importance of the early stage knowledge transfer and the development of these core competencies, many institutions both in the UK and USA have developed or are developing both undergraduate and graduate curricula with a focus on bioinformatics, biotechnology and the interplay between the two. Whilst concerns over course content are, however, important for attracting and educating skilful chemists (Price & Hill, 2004), arguably the greater threat to medicinal and synthetic organic chemistry is funding. It is vital that both industry and academia work with public funding bodies to ensure that the core disciplines that will provide the next generation of innovative and skilled medicinal chemists are appropriately supported at the public, corporate and government level (Pors *et al*, 2009).

3.2 R&D in the emerging markets: An opportunity for collaboration and innovation?

The uncertainty of the funding climate and the lack of innovation (as measured by number of NMEs being approved for market) have naturally given cause for concern. In contrast to what has happened in the western countries after the recession, it appears that emerging markets are on the rise, partly because of heavy investment by the largest pharmaceutical companies in countries such as China over the past decade. Principally, the significantly lower cost of research in emerging economies has lead to a substantial increase in the outsourcing of the more routine activities such as compound synthesis and preclinical toxicity tests, but also outsourcing of R&D to augment internal capabilities of pharmaceutical companies are on the rise (Tremblay, 2010). Besides China, the pharmaceutical companies have used considerable efforts in establishing themselves in the emerging markets including China, India, Brazil, Russia, South Korea and Mexico. Given that 85% of the world's population lives in these countries combined with more open policies has meant that R&D has accelerated enormously in these countries. In 2004, China was the fastest-growing pharmaceutical market with growth rates of 28%. In 2015 Asia is expected to overtake Europe in pharmaceutical sales and become the second largest pharmaceutical market after the United States (Hughes, 2010). By 2050, Asia is projected to be the largest pharmaceutical market (Ward, 2008), which will have significant impact on drug discovery as a whole. The growth of the Chinese health-care market is largely being driven by the changing age profile of the population, its rapid economic development, and urbanization (Ward, 2008). As a consequence, the disease profile in China is changing. For example, type 2 diabetes was a rare disease in China 20 years ago, but its commonness has doubled in the past decade, with more than 55 million people affected today. A recent study conducted from June 2007 to May 2008 reported that 9.7% of the general adult population in China has diabetes and 15.5% have pre-diabetes, compared with 2.4% and 3.2%, respectively, in a similar study in 1994 (Yang *et al*, 2010). This increase in disease incidence has been ascribed to longer life expectancy and lifestyle changes that have occurred through rapid economic growth in especially Asia. As the emerging markets grow, an appreciation of population factors and changes associated with modernization is vital to dealing with and predicting how the Chinese health-care market will evolve (Ward, 2008). This is already starting to impact early-stage research aimed at specific medical needs of patients in these regions but also clinical trials are initiated with focus on enrolling enough patients from central as well as remote regions of China. Both early-stage research and clinical trials are of huge interest to the pharmaceutical industry that is investing heavily in Asia. Current discussion also concerns whether the focus of medical research is directly applicable for patient populations in Asia (Hughes, 2010). China has an estimated 100 million people suffering from hypertension and, with 62% of males being smokers, the country's lung cancer rates are among the highest in the world (Hughes, 2010). India, the second largest populated country in the world with over a billion citizens, has also seen an increase in lifestyle-associated diseases. By 2025, there will be more than 185 million people over the age of 60 years in India. As is often the case with an elderly population there is an increased risk of developing diabetes, cardiovascular disease and maybe also region specific diseases. As a result it is important to think of the medicines that will be available for these countries with regard to the types of disease, as well as their cost and accessibility (Hughes, 2010).

Despite of the investment in the emerging markets, recent data show that the US remains the single-largest location of pharmaceutical invention (Friedman, 2010). They also show that while the established pharmaceutical countries remain strong, there is little measurable innovative activity in terms of NMEs from India or China between 2001 and 2009. However, the factual situation is probably somewhat different due to a substantial time lag of 10 years or more between the initial discovery of a potential drug and its market approval. Indeed, China became the world leader in 2009 in terms of the number of chemistry patents published on an annual basis, according to Chemical Abstracts Service (CAS), a division of the American Chemical Society (Rovner, 2010). Accordingly, the recent nature of the increase in investment in innovative research in China and other emerging countries (Friedman, 2010) could facilitate an opportunity to innovate in a number of areas and as a result lead to a higher number of NMEs for market approval in the future. As such, the outlook for the patient is clearly very exciting. The next 50 years could see joint efforts between established and emerging markets in advancing many industries and technologies including drug discovery. The strategic planning and the vision by the pharmaceutical industry and American and European governments would facilitate a continuous input from established markets with R&D expertise that would maintain a high level of leadership in innovation, but also enable the emerging markets to be key players in future innovation.

4. Future directions

"Prediction is very difficult, especially about the future." Niels Bohr (1885 – 1962)

Drug discovery has come a long way since Paul Ehrlich's research into dyes for medicinal properties. Drug discovery now requires a multidisciplinary effort and the continuing need for the education of excellent scientists working at the interface of chemistry and biology is imperative, not only to successful drug development, but also to the exploration of new targets using small molecules to probe cellular and molecular mechanisms. Indeed, small molecules designed and synthesised in chemistry laboratories have been shown to be valuable for treating diseases and constitute many of the medicines marketed today (Nielsen & Schreiber, 2008a). Consequently, their effect on biomedical research during the past decade has been dramatic, providing both new tools for understanding living systems as well as enabling a didactic transition from biology to medicine (Dobson, 2004; Nielsen & Schreiber, 2008a; Stockwell, 2004). The foundation of HTS technologies, the availability of chem- and bioinformatic databases coupled with emerging tools such as FBDD, DOS and chemical genetics has led drug discovery into the 21st century with optimism for further advancement and understanding of what is required for successful drug development. We know that there is no "magic bullet" around the corner, but through hard work and innovative thinking we are likely improve our knowledge and slowly but incrementally develop better drugs. There must also be an element of braveness and entrepreneurship if we are to solve challenging targets and there is a need for industry and governmental organisations to finance such ventures. For example, ventures into underexploited regions of chemical space is to expand the range of 'druggable' targets, such that the identification of new ligands for currently challenging targets such as protein-protein interaction (Fuller *et al*, 2009) ultimately becomes routine. Success in this endeavour is likely to have major positive impacts in medicinal chemistry, chemical biology and drug discovery (Moura-Letts *et al*, 2011). It is worth noting, however, that the commercial success of a drug is not related to the novelty of the mechanism upon which it is based, but the differentiation that it provides (Booth & Zemmel, 2003; Ma *et al*, 2008). Finding a new therapeutically relevant target is extremely difficult and pioneering drug discovery has become prohibitively expensive. Many validated targets should also be further exploited alongside innovative initiatives to provide better products with lower risk and cost (Zhao & Guo, 2009).

However, there is cause for concern. Declining government funding and reformed educational policies in the western world are likely to have serious implications for drug discovery educators and practitioners, which could widen the already significant gap between research scientists at the highest level and the education of students at undergraduate and postgraduate level. There is a real concern that the scientists of tomorrow will not possess the 'right' tools in the toolkit to be able to effectively interrogate and address the questions being asked by research scientists in academia and industry today. The challenges can only be met if the government agencies worldwide are willing to invest in the education of academics and students alike. The onus is also on academics to be able to adapt to the rapidly changing funding priorities (Pors *et al*, 2009). In addition, drug discovery is entering a period of uncertainty where it is vital that opportunities in the emerging markets are grasped by the horn. A close collaboration between the pharmaceutical industry, governments in US and Europe and the emerging markets is essential for adapting to ever-increasing costs of drug discovery. Accordingly, the recent nature of the increase in investment in innovative research in China and other emerging countries could facilitate an opportunity to innovate in a number of areas and as a result lead to a higher number of NMEs for market approval. The next 50 years could see joint efforts between established and emerging markets in advancing drug discovery. The strategic planning and the vision by the pharmaceutical industry and American and European governments would facilitate a continuous input from established markets with R&D expertise that would maintain a high level of leadership in innovation, but also enable the emerging markets to be key players in future innovation.

5. Acknowledgements

This work was supported by Yorkshire Cancer Research (U.K.). The author is grateful to Dr Robert A. Falconer for critical analysis and useful discussions during manuscript writing. Cheryl S. James is thanked for proofreading of manuscript.

6. References

Abad-Zapatero, C. (2007). A Sorcerer's apprentice and the rule of five: from rule-of-thumb to commandment and beyond. *Drug Discovery Today*, Vol. 12, pp. 995-997

Angell, M. (2004). The Truth About the Drug Companies: How They Deceive Us and What to Do About It pp. Random House Publishing, ISBN 0-37576094-37576096, New York, U.S.

Bauer, R. A.; Wurst J. M. & Tan D. S. (2010). Expanding the range of 'druggable' targets with natural product-based libraries: an academic perspective. *Current Opinion in Chemical Biology*, Vol. 14, pp. 308-314

Bender, A.; Fergus S.; Galloway W. R. J. D.; et al. (2006). Diversity oriented synthesis: A challenge for synthetic chemists. *Chemical Genomics: Small Molecule Probes to Study Cellular Function*, Vol. 58, pp. 47-60

Billingsley, M. L. (2008). Druggable targets and targeted drugs: enhancing the development of new therapeutics. *Pharmacology*, Vol. 82, pp. 239-244

Boehringer, M.; Boehm H. J.; Bur D.; et al. (2000). Novel inhibitors of DNA gyrase: 3D structure based biased needle screening, hit validation by biophysical methods, and 3D guided optimization. A promising alternative to random screening. *Journal of Medicinal Chemistry*, Vol. 43, pp. 2664-2674

Bon, R. S. & Waldmann H. (2010). Bioactivity-guided navigation of chemical space. *Account of Chemical Research*, Vol. 43, pp. 1103-1114

Booth, B. & Zemmel R. (2003). Opinion - Quest for best. *Nature Reviews Drug Discovery*, Vol. 2, pp. 838-841

Brown, J. M. & Wilson W. R. (2004). Exploiting tumour hypoxia in cancer treatment. *Nat Rev Cancer*, Vol. 4, pp. 437-447

Burke, M. (2011). Innovation: Europe must do better. *Chemistry World*, Vol. 8, pp. 12

Burke, M. D. & Schreiber S. L. (2004). A planning strategy for diversity-oriented synthesis. *Angewandte Chemie-International Edition*, Vol. 43, pp. 46-58

Chessari, G. & Woodhead A. J. (2009a). From fragment to clinical candidate--a historical perspective. *Drug Discov Today*, Vol. 14, pp. 668-675

Chessari, G. & Woodhead A. J. (2009b). From fragment to clinical candidate--a historical perspective. *Drug Discovery Today*, Vol. 14, pp. 668-675

Crow, J. M. (2008). UK chemists warn of funding crisis. *In: Chemistry World*, Vol. 5, pp. Available from
http://www.rsc.org/chemistryworld/News/2008/October/20100801.asp

de Kloe, G. E.; Bailey D.; Leurs R.; et al. (2009). Transforming fragments into candidates: small becomes big in medicinal chemistry. *Drug Discov Today*, Vol. 14, pp. 630-646

Denny, W. A. (2002). The contribution of synthetic organic chemistry to anticancer drug development. *In Anticancer Drug Development, (Baguely B.C and Kerr D.J., eds)*, pp. 187-202, Academic Press

Dobson, C. M. (2004). Chemical space and biology. *Nature*, Vol. 432, pp. 824-828

Edwards, P. D.; Albert J. S.; Sylvester M.; et al. (2007). Application of fragment-based lead generation to the discovery of novel, cyclic amidine beta-secretase inhibitors with nanomolar potency, cellular activity, and high ligand efficiency. *Journal of Medicinal Chemistry*, Vol. 50, pp. 5912-5925

European Research Council (2011). ERC Starting Independent Researcher Grant pp. Available at
  http://erc.europa.eu/index.cfm?fuseaction=page.display&topicID=65

Extance, A. (2011). EPSRC plans represent 'huge change'. *Chemistry World*, Vol. 8, p. 8

Feher, M. & Schmidt J. M. (2003). Property distributions: Differences between drugs, natural products, and molecules from combinatorial chemistry. *Journal of Chemical Information and Computer Sciences*, Vol. 43, pp. 218-227

Frantz, S. (2003). Creating the right chemistry. *Nat Rev Drug Discov*, Vol. 2, p. 163

Friedman, Y. (2010). Location of pharmaceutical innovation: 2000-2009. *Nature Reviews Drug Discovery*, Vol. 9, pp. 835-836

Fuller, J. C.; Burgoyne N. J. & Jackson R. M. (2009). Predicting druggable binding sites at the protein-protein interface. *Drug Discovery Today*, Vol. 14, pp. 155-161

Gedye, R.; Smith F.; Westaway K.; et al. (1986). The Use of Microwave-Ovens for Rapid Organic-Synthesis. *Tetrahedron Letters*, Vol. 27, pp. 279-282

Goodman, L. S.; Wintrobe M. M.; Damescheck W.; et al. (1946). Nitrogen mustard therapy. Use of methyl-bis(β-chloroethyl)amine hydrochloride and tris-(β-chloroethyl)amine hydrochloride for Hodgkin's disease, lymphosarcoma, leukemia and certain allied and miscellaneous disorders. *J Am Med Assoc*, Vol. 132, pp. 126-132

Haggarty, S. J.; Koeller K. M.; Wong J. C.; et al. (2003). Multidimensional chemical genetic analysis of diversity-oriented synthesis-derived deacetylase inhibitors using cell-based assays. *Chemical Biology*, Vol. 10, pp. 383-396

Hanson, P. R.; Rolfe A. & Lushington G. H. (2010). Reagent based DOS: A "Click, Click, Cyclize" strategy to probe chemical space. *Organic & Biomolecular Chemistry*, Vol. 8, pp. 2198-2203

Hirsch, J. (2006). An anniversary for cancer chemotherapy. *JAMA*, Vol. 296, pp. 1518-1520

Hopkins, A. L. & Groom C. R. (2002). The druggable genome. *Nature Reviews Drug Discovery*, Vol. 1, pp. 727-730

Hughes, B. (2010). Evolving R&D for emerging markets. *Nature Reviews Drug Discovery*, Vol. 9, pp. 417-420

Justice, B. A.; Badr N. A. & Felder R. A. (2009). 3D cell culture opens new dimensions in cell-based assays. *Drug Discov Today*, Vol. 14, pp. 102-107

Lam, K. S. & Renil M. (2002). From combinatorial chemistry to chemical microarray. *Current Opinion in Chemical Biology*, Vol. 6, pp. 353-358

Lehar, J.; Stockwell B. R.; Giaever G.; et al. (2008a). Combination chemical genetics. *Nature Chemical Biology*, Vol. 4, pp. 674-681

Lehar, J.; Stockwell B. R.; Giaever G.; et al. (2008b). Combination chemical genetics. *Nat Chem Biol*, Vol. 4, pp. 674-681

Lewcock, A. (2009). EPSRC turnaround on blacklisting policy. *Chemistry World*, Vol. 6, pp. Available from
  http://www.rsc.org/chemistryworld/News/2009/May/05050904.asp

Lian, M. (2005). Chemistry education in china. *Nachrichten Aus Der Chemie*, Vol. 53, pp. 622-627

Lipinski, C. A.; Lombardo F.; Dominy B. W.; et al. (1997). Experimental and computational approaches to estimate solubility and permeability in drug discovery and development settings. *Advanced Drug Delivery Reviews*, Vol. 23, pp. 3-25

Lombardino, J. G. & Lowe J. A., 3rd (2004). The role of the medicinal chemist in drug discovery--then and now. *Nat Rev Drug Discov*, Vol. 3, pp. 853-862

Ma, P.; Gudiksen M.; Fleming E.; et al. (2008). Outlook - What drives success for specialty pharmaceuticals? *Nature Reviews Drug Discovery*, Vol. 7, pp. 563-567

Moos, W. H.; Hurt C. R. & Morales G. A. (2009). Combinatorial chemistry: oh what a decade or two can do. *Molecular Diversity*, Vol. 13, pp. 241-245

Moura-Letts, G.; Diblasi C. M.; Bauer R. A.; et al. (2011). Solid-phase synthesis and chemical space analysis of a 190-membered alkaloid/terpenoid-like library. *Proc Natl Acad Sci U S A*, Vol. 108, pp. 6745-6750

Mullin, R. (2010). Battening the Hatches. *Chemical & Engineering News*, Vol. 88, p. 14

Munos, B. (2009). Lessons from 60 years of pharmaceutical innovation. *Nature Reviews Drug Discovery*, Vol. 8, pp. 959-968

National Cancer Institute (2011a). Cancer Research Funding. pp. Available at http://www.cancer.gov/cancertopics/factsheet/NCI/research-funding

National Cancer Institute (2011b). The NCI Budget in Review. pp. Available at http://obf.cancer.gov/financial/factbook.htm

Nghiem, P. & Kawasumi M. (2007). Chemical genetics: Elucidating biological systems with small-molecule compounds. *Journal of Investigative Dermatology*, Vol. 127, pp. 1577-1584

Nielsen, T. E. & Schreiber S. L. (2008a). Towards the optimal screening collection: a synthesis strategy. *Angew Chem Int Ed Engl*, Vol. 47, pp. 48-56

Nielsen, T. E. & Schreiber S. L. (2008b). Towards the optimal screening collection: a synthesis strategy. *Angewandte Chemie-International Edition*, Vol. 47, pp. 48-56

Overington, J. P.; Al-Lazikani B. & Hopkins A. L. (2006). Opinion - How many drug targets are there? *Nature Reviews Drug Discovery*, Vol. 5, pp. 993-996

Philpott, K. L.; Hughes J. P.; Rees S.; et al. (2011). Principles of early drug discovery. *British Journal of Pharmacology*, Vol. 162, pp. 1239-1249

Pittman, D. (2010). Changing Their Ways. *Chemical & Engineering News*, Vol. 88, pp. 47-49

Pors, K.; Goldberg F. W.; Leamon C. P.; et al. (2009). The changing landscape of cancer drug discovery: a challenge to the medicinal chemist of tomorrow. *Drug Discovery Today*, Vol. 14, pp. 1045-1050

Price, W. S. & Hill J. O. (2004). Raising the Status of Chemistry Education. *The Royal Society of Chemistry*, pp. 13-20

Reymond, J. L. & Fink T. (2007). Virtual exploration of the chemical universe up to 11 atoms of C, N, O, F: Assembly of 26.4 million structures (110.9 million stereoisomers) and analysis for new ring systems, stereochemistry, physicochemical properties, compound classes, and drug discovery. *Journal of Chemical Information and Modeling*, Vol. 47, pp. 342-353

Rooseboom, M.; Commandeur J. N. & Vermeulen N. P. (2004). Enzyme-catalyzed activation of anticancer prodrugs. *Pharmacol Rev*, Vol. 56, pp. 53-102

Rovner, S. L. (2010). China Ascendant. *Chemical & Engineering News*, Vol. 88, pp. 35-37

Rydzewski, R. M. (2008). The Drug Discovery Busines to Date. *In: Real World Drug Discovery: A Chemist's Guide to Biotech and Pharmaceutical Research*, pp. 1-52, Elsevier, ISBN: 978-970-908-046617-046610, Amsterdam, The Netherlands.

SalimiMoosavi, H.; Tang T. & Harrison D. J. (1997). Electroosmotic pumping of organic solvents and reagents in microfabricated reactor chips. *Journal of the American Chemical Society*, Vol. 119, pp. 8716-8717

Sharpless, K. B.; Kolb H. C. & Finn M. G. (2001). Click chemistry: Diverse chemical function from a few good reactions. *Angewandte Chemie-International Edition*, Vol. 40, pp. 2004-2021

Shoichet, B. K.; Hert J.; Irwin J. J.; et al. (2009). Quantifying biogenic bias in screening libraries. *Nature Chemical Biology*, Vol. 5, pp. 479-483

Sneader, W. E. (2005). Legacy of the past. *Drug discovery: a history*, pp. John Wiley & Sons Ltd, ISBN-10 10-471-89979-89978, West Sussex (U.K.)

Spandl, R. J.; Bender A. & Spring D. R. (2008). Diversity-oriented synthesis; a spectrum of approaches and results. *Organic & Biomolecular Chemistry*, Vol. 6, pp. 1149-1158

Spring, D. R.; Spandl R. J. & Bender A. (2008). Diversity-oriented synthesis; a spectrum of approaches and results. *Organic & Biomolecular Chemistry*, Vol. 6, pp. 1149-1158

Stockwell, B. R. (2004). Exploring biology with small organic molecules. *Nature*, Vol. 432, pp. 846-854

Strebhardt, K. & Ullrich A. (2008). Paul Ehrlich's magic bullet concept: 100 years of progress. *Nature Reviews Cancer*, Vol. 8, pp. 473-480

Studer, A.; Hadida S.; Ferritto R.; et al. (1997). Fluorous synthesis: A fluorous-phase strategy for improving separation efficiency in organic synthesis. *Science*, Vol. 275, pp. 823-826

Swinney, D. C. & Anthony J. (2011). How were new medicines discovered? *Nature Reviews Drug Discovery*, Vol. 10, pp. 507-519

Tralau-Stewart, C. J.; Wyatt C. A.; Kleyn D. E.; et al. (2009). Drug discovery: new models for industry-academic partnerships. *Drug Discov Today*, Vol. 14, pp. 95-101

Tremblay, J. F. (2010). The Grand Experiment. *Chemical & Engineering News*, Vol. 88, p. 20

U.S. Department of Health & Human Services (2010). Research Project and R01-equivalent grants: success rates of new applications, by submission number. pp. Available at http://report.nih.gov/success_rates/index.aspx

Ward, S. (2008). Demographic factors in the Chinese health-care market. *Nature Reviews Drug Discovery*, Vol. 7, pp. 383-384

Wilhelm, S.; Carter C.; Lynch M.; et al. (2006). Discovery and development of sorafenib: a multikinase inhibitor for treating cancer. *Nature Reviews Drug Discovery*, Vol. 5, pp. 835-844

Yang, S. H.; Dou K. F. & Song W. J. (2010). Prevalence of diabetes among men and women in China. *New England Journal of Medicine*, Vol. 362, pp. 2425-2426; author reply 2426

Zamir, E. & Bastiaens P. I. H. (2008). Reverse engineering intracellular biochemical networks. *Nature Chemical Biology*, Vol. 4, pp. 643-647

Zartler, E. R. & Shapiro M. J. (2005). Fragonomics: fragment-based drug discovery. *Current Opinion in Chemical Biology*, Vol. 9, pp. 366-370

Zhao, H. & Guo Z. (2009). Medicinal chemistry strategies in follow-on drug discovery. *Drug Discov Today*, Vol. 14, pp. 516-522

Zlokarnik, G.; Grootenhuis P. D. & Watson J. B. (2005). High throughput P450 inhibition screens in early drug discovery. *Drug Discov Today*, Vol. 10, pp. 1443-1450

3

Drug Discovery and Ayurveda: Win-Win Relationship Between Contemporary and Ancient Sciences

Bhushan Patwardhan[1] and Kapil Khambholja[2]
[1]*Symbiosis International University, Pune,*
[2]*Novartis Healthcare Pvt. Limited, Hyderabad,*
India

1. Introduction

The present medicinal system is dominated by the Allopathy or western medicine which is prominently taught and practiced in most of the countries world wide. This system is still evolving and during last few decades focus was based on chemical origin of most of the medicines. Thus majority of drugs in current practice are from synthetic origin. Even so, a large number of these synthetic molecules are based directly or indirectly on natural products or phytoconstituents (Gupta *et al.* 2005; Harvey 2008) . The interesting question is – what type of medicines were people using for thousands of decades? Another interesting futuristic question is – What type of medicine / therapy would emerge and sustain in future? Answers to such questions can be obtained by doing a systemic review of existing scientific literature and also by making a forecast based on emerging technologies based on genetic sciences. Another important arena of brainstorming is how we link such questions with each other. We need to understand medicines or systems those were existing in use before emergence of current "synthetic era" and visualize the future of medicine and health care in the "technology era". The linkage between "the past" and "the future" of medicine is much more important and can give us "new directions" for better understanding health, disease and possible solutions.

Ayurveda, one of the oldest systems used by mankind for well being(Sharma 1995), originated in ancient India many thousand years ago (about 4500 BC as agreed by most scientists). The origin, development, existence and even practice of Ayurveda has many dimensions and complex theories based on religions, faith and ancient Vedic science (Patwardhan & Mashelkar 2009). Discussion on all these aspects is beyond the scope of this book chapter. Ayurveda, as a system of medicine, is one of the official systems of medicine in India (Mashelkar 2008) and is also widely practiced in many other countries (Mashelkar 2008). Evidence for effectiveness of many ayurvedic drugs and therapies is being generated rapidly from many research institutes and also there are projects under way to decipher unanswered questions related to Ayurveda. In this chapter we have tried to cover different but important aspects which give us a futuristic vision. After giving an overview of basics of Ayurveda, a comprehensive review of current status of research in Ayurveda is attempted. In later part of the chapter a dialogue on the key term "Drug Rediscovery" is being presented for the first time with a scientific perspective. The later part of the chapter also covers futuristic discussion where possibilities of linking Ayurveda with drug discovery process are described. We have tried to lay down conceptual framework for win-win relationship between ancient and contemporary health care sciences backed by strong scientific evidence being generated in recent years. We hope to provide innovative material for use in further development by scientific fraternity for ultimate benefit of health care and humanity.

1.1 Introduction to Ayurveda
There exist a plethora of information on Ayurveda through many books and commentaries published in past few decades. Most of these books are based on the traditional books which are thought to carry the knowledge and know-how of Ayurveda which, in ancient time, was existing in the form of memorised shlokas and manuscripts written in Sanskrit language. In this part of the chapter we have tried to present brief and comprehensive introduction to Ayurveda and its' fundamentals. The information provided is just a drop in the ocean and represents only that which is relevant to understanding the concept of Ayurveda and its further use in drug discovery process.

1.2 What is Ayurveda?
Ayurveda literally means "science of life" in Sanskrit (Ayur: Life; Veda: Science). It is not only a medical system but a way of life. As discussed earlier Ayurveda aims at a holistic management of health and diseases. It is widely practiced in the Indian subcontinent and is also one of the official systems of medicine in India. Its concepts and approaches are considered to have been perfected between 2500-500 BC.

Charak Samhita and *Sushrut Samhita* (100-500 BC) are the two main Ayurvedic classics, wherein more than 700 plants along with their classification, pharmacological and therapeutic properties have been described. Ayurveda during course of ancient times developed as sound scientific system and it is evident as it is divided into eight major disciplines known as *Ashtanga Ayurveda*. It is important to note that these specialisations or super specialisations were in existence and practiced by experts hundreds of years before the emergence of modern Anatomy, physiology and contemporary medicinal system!

1.3 Fundamentals and perspectives
1.3.1 Ashtanga Ayurveda: Specialities of knowledge in Ayurveda
Eight major divisions of Ayurveda have been described and followed for specialized knowledge. These categories are:
1. Kayachikistsa : The closest synonym would be internal medicine,
2. Shalya: General Surgery,
3. Shalakya: Speciality dealing with head and neck disorders,
4. Kaumar-bhritya: obstetrics and pediatrics
5. Rasayana: geriatrics and rejuvenative/reparative medicine
6. Vajikaran: Sexology and reproductive medicine,
7. Agad-Tantra: the body of knowledge on poisons, venoms and toxic substances,
8. Bhuta-Vidya: infectious diseases and mental illness. The fact that such a systemic categorization was established so early speaks of the knowledge and skills being central to the practice of Ayurveda.

Another fundamental concept of Ayurveda is the well defined system for classifying the individuals on basis of their body constitution, physiology and other relevant factors. The concept of "Prakruti" is thought to be at the base of many important steps in Ayurvedic diagnosis and therapy.

Prakriti is a consequence of the relative proportion of three entities (Tri-Doshas), Vata (V), Pitta (P) and Kapha (K), which are not only genetically determined (Shukra Shonita), but also influenced by environment (Mahabhuta Vikara), maternal diet and lifestyle (Matur Ahara Vihara), and age of the transmitting parents (Kala -Garbhashaya).

In an individual, the Tri-Doshas work in conjunction and maintain homeostasis throughout the lifetime starting from fertilization. Distinct properties and functions have been ascribed to each Dosha. For instance, Vata contributes to manifestation of shape, cell division, signaling, movement, excretion of wastes, cognition and also regulates the activities of Kapha and Pitta. Kapha is responsible for anabolism, growth and maintenance of structure, storage and stability. Pitta is primarily responsible for metabolism, thermo-regulation, energy homeostasis, pigmentation, vision, and host surveillance.

1.4 Drugs of Ayurveda

Drugs used in Ayurvdea are mostly herbs (crude or processed), minerals products, metals (in different oxidised forms prepared by specialised manufacturing techniques) and also some times animal products. It is to be noted that in many instances a combination of one or more of above type of drugs are prescribed. As per Ayurveda- drugs alone cannot fulfil the goal of achieving, improving or maintaining the healthy state of the body. The lifestyle, food habits, environment and more importantly the mind plays an important role in Health. Thus the Vaidya (Ayurvedic physician) suggests a complete regime which is composed of a set of ayurvedic drugs (herbs/ herbo-mineral formulations) to be taken in specified manner in combination of food and life style changes are to be followed strictly, to achieve a healthy state of mind and body.

In last few years lots of research has been undertaken on medicinal properties, possible mechanisms and other relevant information on many popular herbs mentioned in traditional texts and used by Vaidyas. These research projects, mainly pre-clinical studies, help to generate evidence behind ayurvedic drugs' clinical use. Many interesting leads are emerging for further drug discovery from Ayurvedic drugs (Patawardhan et al. 2004,). These contributions are sometimes forgotten in the current dominance of the reductionist paradigm. Table 1 enlists some of the Ayurvedic herbs, which have been widely used and subject to pharmacological research. The structural modifications of active principles of these plants have led to a plethora of new "chemical" drugs and still there exist a vast unexplored arena for SAR based studies which may lead to unique molecules with unprecedented safety and efficacy. Since many decades several of these plants are being globally used by thousands of licensed Vaidyas and other practitioners and even as a part of household tradition. Looking into this background it is desirable to understand the Ayurvedic properties of herbs. This approach would assist in evolving innovative combinations, investigate new uses and conduct clinical trials with appropriate targets. As for example, a judicious and standardized combination of Aloe vera gel and Curcuma longa rhizome powder may yield a potent wound and burn healing new product. Similarly, a combination of Glycyrrhiza glabra and Zingiber officinale would be more useful in acid-peptic disease than the single ingredients. But any such combination must have a rational Ayurvedic basis, rather than herbal concoctions. Understanding the ayurvedic basis of any combination of herbs and its use in different condition requires knowledge of ayurvedic fundamentals and its correlation with contemporary concepts. Table 1 represent some examples of current evidence for ayurvedic drugs and their untapped potential yet to be established extending their scientific basis from Ayurveda (Vaidya AB 2006).

For further information and detailed knowledge readers are advised to study following subjects / specialisations of Ayurveda.

1.5 Ayurvedic pharmaceuticals

Bhaisajya Kalpana (Ayurvedic Pharmaceutics) forms a branch of Ayurveda, which mainly deals with collection and selection of ayurvedic drugs, purification as well as preparation, preservation, besides mode of administration and dosage specification. The ancient Ayurvedic scholars were very much rational and had a strong scientific background in fundamental principles, which are concerned with drug manufacturing.

Dravyagunavigyana includes identification (pharmacognosy-Namarupa vigyanya), preparation (pharmacy-Kalpa Vigyana) and administration (clinical pharmacology-Yoga Vigyana). The later deals with the effects of drugs on various systems (pharmacodynamics-Gunakarma Vigyana) and their application in different diseases (therapeutic-Pryoga Vigyana)

Ayurvedic Plant	Impact	Untapped potential
Aloe vera	Cosmetopharmaocolgy/ Burns	Menopause/Andropause
Atropa belladona	Acetyl choline pharmacology	Cigarrete for asthama
Azadirachta indica	Antiinsect/Antifungal	Head and neck cancer
Cassia angustifolia	Laxative/Indigetion	Chronic infections
Curcuma longa	Antiinflammatory/Antidiabetic	Cancer
Commiphora wightii	Antiarthritic/Obesity	Tuberculosis/Anti cancer
Glycyrrhiza glabra	Peptic ulcer/Sore throat	Anti viral/Anti cancer
Psoralea coryllifolia	Leucoderma/Psoriasis	Antimicrobial/Alopecia
Rauwolfia serpentina	Antihypertensive/tranquillizer	Antivenom
Strychnos nux-vomica	Digestive/Nervine tonic	Glycinergic receptors
Tinospora cordifolia	Immuostimulant/Anticancer	Hepatoprotective
Withania somnifera	Sedative/Phytoestrogen	Anticancer
Zingiber officinalis	Indigetion/Nausea	Arthritis

Table 1. Ayurvedic plants and impact on therapy and drug discovery

2. Contemporary drug discovery / development research on Ayurvedic concepts and medicines

As discussed above Ayurvedic concepts differ significantly when it comes to diagnosis, use of drugs or even treatment pedagogy. It is well-known that Ayurveda tries to heal or cure any disease condition from its grass-root level. It means, it does not only remove the symptoms of the condition, but also alleviates the cause or factors behind the disease. In this part of the chapter we would share and discuss few examples of research done on ayurvedic concepts and medicines using contemporary technologies or methodologies.

2.1 Exploring targets - Understanding mechanisms
There are many studies reported where preclinical or even clinical evidence has been generated for understanding targets or even mechanisms for Ayurvedic therapies. Another important aspect of research is to correlate ayurvedic fundamentals behind etiology, disease progression and its possible interventions in terms of contemporary medical/life science.

2.2 Correlating ancient science with contemporary pathophysiology and medicinal system
An article published by Sharma and Chandola, discusses the details of "Prameha" of Ayurveda and its correlation with obesity, metabolic syndrome, and diabetes mellitus (Sharma& Chandola 2011). The authors have given scientific basis of correlation and have described etiology, classification, and pathogenesis of these conditions both in terms of ayurvedic and modern concepts. According to this article there are 20 subtypes of Prameha due to the interaction of the three Doshas and 10 Dushyas (disturbed functioning of the principles that support the various bodily tissues); several of these subtypes have sweet urine, whereas some of them have different coloration of the urine, highlighting the inflammatory conditions involved in the metabolic syndrome. This disease has close ties to Sthaulya (i.e., obesity). With regard to diabetes mellitus, Sahaja Prameha and Jatah Pramehi correlate with type 1 diabetes; Apathyanimittaja Pramehacorrelates with type 2 diabetes. Madhumeha is a subtype of Vataja Prameha (Prameha withVata predominance) that can occur as the terminal stage of type 2 diabetes (in which insulin is required), or as type 1 diabetes beginning in early childhood. The latter is defined as Jatah Pramehi Madhumehino in Charaka Samhita, one of the classical Ayurvedic texts. The authors have concluded that various dietary, lifestyle, and psychologic factors are involved in the etiology of Prameha, particularly in relation to disturbances in fat and carbohydrate metabolism. The ancient Ayurvedic knowledge regarding Prameha can be utilized to expand the current understanding of obesity, metabolic syndrome, and diabetes.

2.3 Discovery through pre-clinical studies for understanding mechanism and targets for Ayurvedic drugs
As discussed earlier there are many papers being published regularly in national and international journals which provide evidence based on pre clinical studies and also some times provide probable mechanism of the ayurvedic drug / formulation under study. Few such examples are quoted here to reiterate the fact that ayurvedic drugs and therapies are having sound scientific background and one of the primary things remaining is to generate evidence so as to understand their utility and mechanism from contemporary science's point of view. In 2009 our team published results for understanding the immunomodulatory effect of "Shatavri" (*Asparagus racemosus*). Shatavri is one of the reputed and widely used rasayana herb of Ayurveda and is responsible for providing rejevunating effect along with other beneficial effects. In this article mixed Th1/Th2 activity of shatavri extracts is proven supporting its immunoadjuvant potential (Gautam *et al.* 2009).

In another mechanistic study Chondroprotective potential of Extracts of Almalki Fruits *(Phyllanthus emblica)* in Osteoarthritis was undertaken to understand mechanism behind the traditional use of Almalki. Chondroprotection was measured in three different assay systems. First, the effects of fruit powder were studied on the activities of the enzymes hyaluronidase and collagenase type 2. Second, an in vitro model of cartilage degradation was set-up with explant cultures of articular knee cartilage from osteoarthritis patients. Cartilage damage was assayed by measuring glycosaminoglycan release from explants treated with/without *P. emblica* fruit powders. Aqueous extracts of both fruit powders significantly inhibited the activities of hyaluronidase and collagenase type 2 in vitro. Third, in the explant model of cartilage matrix damage, extracts of glucosamine sulphate and selected extract exhibited statistically significant, long-term chondroprotective activity in cartilage explants from 50% of the patients tested (Sumantran *et al.* 2008).

2.4 Clinical evidence for medicinal uses of Ayurvedic drugs

Apart from pre-clinical studies many clinical studies of various depths are also being reported recently. Additionally the Government of India supported Department of AYUSH undertakes many clinical research based projects on prioritised ayurvedic medicines and formulations. One of the clinical studies we would like to quote here as reference is for studying efficacy of standardised ayurvedic formulation in arthritis. The multidisciplinary "New Millennium Indian Technology Leadership Initiative" Arthritis Project was supported by Government of India. It included randomised controlled exploratory trial with *Zingiber officinale* and *Tinospora cordifoliaas* as main drugs in the formulations under study. Total 245 eligible patients suffering from symptomatic osteo arthritic knees gave consent for it and were randomized into seven arms (35 patients per arm) of a double blind, parallel efficacy, and multicentre drug trial of sixteen weeks duration. The trial was controlled for placebo and glucosamine sulphate use. No dietary or other restrictions were advised. The groups matched well at baseline. There were no differences between the groups for patient withdrawals (total forty three) or adverse events (AE) which were all mild. In an intention-to-treat primary efficacy analysis, there were no significant differences ($P < .05$) for pain (weight bearing) and WOMAC questionnaire (knee function); a high placebo response was recorded. Based on better pain relief, significant ($P < .05$) least analgesic consumption, and improved knee status, one of the formulations under study "C" formulation was selected for further development. This study gives overview suggesting that how the clinical research on ayurvedic herbs or formulations can generate the evidence and also in understanding their possible mechanism of action (Chopra et al. 2011).

2.5 Clinical evidence for Ayurvedic therapy

As discussed earlier most of the time Ayurvedic physicians undertake different approaches for treatment where multiple drugs or formulations are used at one or different stages therapy. One such popular approach in Ayurveda is "Pachkarma therapy" which is used for variety of conditions where detoxification is required to cope up with stress or unbalanced physiology. Ayurvedic drugs or formulations used in such therapy can lead to a very different approach of drug discovery where multiple drugs are working together on multiple targets to achieve the objective of balancing the body physiology.

One such study is reported by Tripathi et al. (2010). This was a comparative clinical trial on the role of Panchakarma therapy and Unmada Gajankusha Rasa in the cases of major depressive disorder vis-à-vis kaphaja Unmada.

2.6 Safety pharmacology and drug interaction studies as part of drug discovery based on ayurvedic drugs

In contemporary Drug discovery programs safety has prime importance and any molecule must have a favorable risk benefit ratio to be considered and approved as drug. Even though ayurvedic drugs and/or formulations are in use by public and vaidyas since antiquities, most of them have a proven record of safety and tolerability. Any change or deviation in method of preparation or use other then that mentioned in traditional text requires additional studies to evaluate safety. Another safety aspect includes understanding of drug interactions if ayurvedic drugs are to be taken with other form of medicines. These sub parts of drug discovery process can be addressed by undertaking invitro toxicology studies and pharmacokinetic studies to understand drug interactions. In one of the studies we have reported Safety Pharmacology and Drug Interaction aspects of *Cassia auriculata*. In this study routine safety pharmacology with focus on cardiovascular variables and pharmacokinetic herb-drug interaction studies on rats fed with standardized traditional hydro-alcoholic extract and technology-based supercritical extract of Cassia auriculata for 12 weeks were undertaken. These studies indicate that both these extracts are pharmacologically safe and did not show any significant adverse reactions at the tested doses. The traditional hydro-alcoholic extract did not show any significant effect on pharmacokinetics; however, the technology-based supercritical extract caused a significant reduction in absorption of Metformin (Puranik et al. 2011).

These and many other such studies describe the way of incorporation of safety aspect in drug discovery process for Ayurvedic drugs.

3. Concept of "Drug rediscovery"

Contemporary Drug discovery and development (DD) process is becoming longer and expensive. Establishing the right balance between efficacy and safety is the crucial part of DD process. As the chemical entity under study would be completely new and no prior human exposure is reported, there are chances of many unexpected side effects being observed at various stages of development. These require multiple efforts for optimisation of the molecule for its safety and efficacy and many times the molecule under study has to be dropped from study due to high toxicity or side effects.

Most ayurvedic drugs / herbs are in use since times immemorable and experience of thousands of physicians is available to vindicate their safety and efficacy. Thus drug discovery process needs to be modified if benefits from Ayurvedic science are to be tapped. Many scholars have previously reported different approaches for this. "Reverse pharmacology" approach starts with clinical studies and goes upto the mechanistic pre-clinical studies (Patwardhan 2004).

Here we deploy a term "Drug rediscovery" which is more relevant for research involving ayurvedic herbs and drugs. As ayurvedic drugs are already in use as part of medicinal system any further research on these drugs would aid only in understanding their mechanisms and / or help in optimising their doses either alone or in combination. Thus the term "Drug rediscovery" would help differentiate process of discovering a drug from totally new chemical entity from the process of understanding a drug which is not totally new to mankind.

Another extension of Drug rediscovery from ayurvedic drugs can be done for benefit of contemporary science of medicine and that would be "stage 2 drug discovery" based on results of research done during drug rediscovery of ayurvedic drugs and herbs. This stage 2 DD would start only after bio-marker based research which is a part of Drug rediscovery of ayurvedic drugs. This may generate to newer leads with multiple targets and can give new direction to speed up the existing discovery path adopted. This concept is explained in Table 2.

Stage I :

DRUG REDISCOVERY on Ayurvedic Drugs

•Proven Ayurvedic drugs to be studied for phytoconstituents
•Activity guided fractionation of Biomarkers
•SAR studies of active constituents
•Mechanistic studies (Preclinical & Clinical)
•**All these leads to optimized therapy based on new evidences to be clubbed with traditional knowledge**

Stage II:

Drug Discovery: Outputs of SAR studies (Stage I) from Ayurvedic Drug rediscovery program

- New LEADS

- Lead optimization and study on new molecule with unique safety and efficacy profile

Outputs of Mechanistic studies of Ayurvedic Drug rediscovery program

• Unique mechanism with multiple targets.
• New target identificaton and validation.
• Systems biology approach potentiating:
  • Single drug / molecule working on multiple targets or even multiple systems.
  • Multi herb-Multi target

Table 2. Unique potential of Ayurvedic Drugs for Drug (Re)discovery

3.1 Accelerated clinical research

The process of rediscovering a drug on basis of its ayurvedic origin involves reverse pharmacology and requires different approaches for undertaking clinical research. One of the approaches can be retrospective study based on hospitals' or clinicians' (vaidya in most of the cases) practice of particular disease or herb. This would be little difficult looking into differences in documentation and record keeping practices in most of the parts of India where Ayurveda is regularly practiced. Another approach for undertaking clinical study can be based on Reverse pharmacology where drug under study can be selected on basis of its clinical use and field experience. We have already discussed one such study earlier in this chapter where randomized, controlled exploratory clinical study on ayurvedic formulation was done for its use in osteoparthritic conditions (Chopra et al. 2011). This study along with standardization of formulation was completed in 23 months and thus the time of generation of evidence is comparatively low as that of contemporary discovery of newer molecules. Even WHO had published guideline mentioning different requirements for clinical research on Traditional medicines (2000). Thus the concepts of "Reverse pharmacology" and "Drug Rediscovery" through Ayurvedic drugs can significantly reduce the time-lag between induction of research project and clinical evidence generation through scientifically designed clinical research.

3.2 AyuGenomis: Role in future of drug discovery

Biotechnology with its specialisations like genomics, proteomics, genetic engineering etc. has made immense advances in deciphering diseases conditions, disease progression, prognosis and even up-to certain level cure for particular conditions. Genomics can play important role both in prevention and treatment of many diseases (Steinberg et al. 2001). The advanced technologies used in genomics and related sciences can help understanding role of genes in diseases and health. The use of these technologies and concepts for generating scientific evidence behind concepts of Ayurveda can open up many interesting avenues.

Structural and functional genetic differences in humans can take the form of single nucleotide polymorphisms (SNP), copy number variations (CNVs), and epigenetic or gene expression modifications. As per current research, in human 99.5 % genetic similarity is found and almost all physiological or anatomical variations amongst person to person are due to 0.5% diversity in single nucleotide polymorphism (SNP) and other variations in nucleotides (Levy *et al.* 2007). These inherited inter-individual variations in DNA sequence contribute to phenotypic variation, influencing an individual's anthropometric characteristics, risk of disease and response to the environment. Characterizing genetic variation may bring improved understanding of differential susceptibility to disease, differential drug response, and the complex interaction of genetic and environmental factors, which go to produce each phenotype.

Ayurveda, the traditional system of Indian medicine, Traditional Chinese medicine and Korean medicine all have well-defined systems of constitutional types used in prescribing medication bearing distinct similarities to contemporary pharmacogenomics. The pharmacognenomics can become useful for understanding genetic basis of concept of "Prakriti". This part of the chapter would discuss about how Pharmacogenomics and Ayurveda can be researched together for unpacking vast possibilities of integrated science.

According to Ayurveda an individual's basic constitution to a large extent determines predisposition and prognosis to diseases as well as therapy and life-style regime. Importance of such individual variations in health and disease is an important basic principle of ayurveda and was underlined by Charaka sometime 4000 years ago as follows:

'Every individual is different from another
and hence should be considered as a different entity.
As many variations are there in the Universe, all are seen in Human being'.
In the Ayurveda system of medicine, predisposition to a disease as well as selection of a preventive and curative regime is primarily based on phenotypic assessment of a person which includes one's body constitution termed "Prakriti". The concept of Prakriti is already discussed in detail earlier in this chapter.

The phenotypic diversity, according to Ayurveda, is a consequence of a continuum of relative proportions of Doshas resulting in seven possible constitutional types namely Vata (V), Pitta(P), Kapha(K), Vata-Pitta, Pitta-Kapha, Vata-Kapha and Vata-Pitta-Kapha. Amongst these, the first three are considered as extremes, exhibiting readily recognizable phenotypes, and are more predisposed to specific diseases.

Better characterization of the human genome has improved the scientific basis for understanding individual variation. The Ayurvedic Prakriti concept should be examined from a genomic perspective. Permutations and combinations of V, P, K attribute characters along with other host factors such as tissue status (Dhatusarata), twenty Gunas, digestive capacity and metabolic power (Agni), psychological nature (Manas Prakriti), habitat (Desha), and season (Kaala), lead to sufficient numbers of variants to define a unique constitution for every individual. Ayurveda thus describes the basis of individual variation(Bhushan 2007).

In the realm of modern predictive medicine, efforts are being directed towards capturing disease phenotypes with greater precision for successful identification of markers for prospective disease conditions.

Ayurveda has been investigated for this purpose, based on the hypothesis that Prakriti types (V, P and K) may offer phenotypic datasets suitable for analysis of underlying genetic variation. As a proof of concept, in the first study done by us, we evaluated 76 subjects both for their Prakriti and HLA DRB1 types, finding significant correlations in support of it (Patwardhan et al. 2005). The study concluded that Ayurveda based phenomes may provide a model to study multigenic traits, possibly offering a new approach to correlating genotypes with phenotypes for human classification.

The three major constitution types described in Ayurveda have unique putative metabolic activities, K being slow, P fast, while V is considered to have variable metabolism. We hypothesized that this might relate to drug metabolism and genetic polymorphism of drug metabolizing enzymes (DME). Inter-individual variability in drug response can be attributed to polymorphism in genes encoding different drug metabolizing enzymes, drug transporters and enzymes involved in DNA biosynthesis and repair. Gene polymorphisms precipitate in different phenotypic subpopulations of drug metabolizer. Poor metabolizers (PM) have high plasma concentration of the drug for longer periods and so retain drugs in the body for longer times. Intermediate metabolizers retain drugs in the body for normal time periods. Extensive metabolizers (EM) retain drugs in the body for the least time, plasma concentrations being high for shorter periods.

In another study we investigated the distribution of drug metabolizing enzymes CYP2C19 and CYP2C9 genotypes in 132 healthy individuals of different Prakriti classes(Ghodke et al. 2009). The results obtained suggest possible association of CYP2C19 gene polymorphism with Prakriti phenotypes.

Overview of few such studies are given in Table No 3 which gives successful lead to new directions for further research.

medicine/intervention	target/enzyme	no. of person	Output	Ref. no
corelation between Human Leucocytes Antigen(HLA) and prakriti type	HLA DRB1 gene	Total 76 person 10 - vata 32 – kapha 34 – pitta prakriti	There is complete absence of HLA DRB1*02 in Vata and HLA DRB1*13 in Kapha	(Bhushan et al. 2005)
correlation between CYP2C19 Gene Polymorphism and prakriti type associated with metabolic activity	CYP2C19 (a variant of the enzyme, cytochrome P450)	132 healthy subjects	The extensive metabolizer (EM) genotype was predominant in Pitta Prakriti (91%), Poor metabolizer (31%) in Kapha Prakriti when compared with Vata (12%) and Pitta Prakriti (9%).	(Ghodke et al. 2009)
Ayurveda's 'Rasa' correspondence with pharmacological activity	Ibuprofen, oleocanthal (from olive oil)		substances' similarities of 'Rasa' may indicate similar pharmacological activity & assumes a new significance to distinguish all the kinds of molecule	(Joshi et al. 2007)
The molecular correlation between the different constitution types	genome wide expression levels, biochemical and hematological parameters, Gene Ontology (GO) and pathway based analysis	Total 96 individuals Vata-39 Pitta-29 Kapha-28	The extreme constitution types revealed differences at gene expression level, biochemical levels. It provide a strong basis for integration of this holistic science with modern genomic approaches for predictive marker discovery and system biology studies.	(Prasher et al. 2008)
EGLN1 involvement in high-altitude adaptation revealed through genetic analysis of extreme constitution types defined in Ayurveda	EGLN1 is a key oxygen sensor gene inhibit hypoxia-inducible factor (HIF-1A).	24 different Indian Populations	TT genotype of rs479200 was more frequent in Kapha types and correlated with higher expression of EGLN1, was associated with patients suffering from high-altitude pulmonary edema, whereas it was present at a significantly lower frequency in Pitta and nearly absent in natives of high altitude.	(Aggarwal et al. 2010)

Table 3. Advanced studies on Ayurvedic fundamentals

Thus it can be summarised that identification of genetic variations underlying metabolic variability in Prakriti may provide newer approach to Pharmacogenomics. Extensive studies on Prakriti subtypes and genome wide single nucleotide polymorphism (SNP) mapping especially of other important DME polymorphisms like CYP2D6, CYP2C9, CYP3A4, TPMT, etc., would be useful to understand possible Prakriti pharmacogenomics relationship correlating genotype, Prakriti and drug metabolism.

Thus, these studies support that Ayurveda Classification is based on genome differentiation and having correlation with different drug responses and adverse effect. The Ayurvedic classification shows similar principle of pharmacogenomics for selecting "right drug, right dosage and to the right patient". There are many such studies required to prove the scientific basis of many of the un-deciphered complex Ayurvedic principles and fundamentals given in Vedic science of life. It seems that thousands of years before, Ayurvedic experts had known effect of genetic variation on physiology and pharmacology much more in details and current scientific tools fell short of understanding such complex concepts of Ayurveda.

An integration of traditional systems of medicine(Ayurveda, TCM, SCM, Kampo) with pharmacogenomics utilizes the advantage of high throughput DNA sequencing, gene mapping, and bioinformatics to identify the actual genetic basis of 'interindividual' and 'interracial' variation in drug efficacy and metabolism and holds promise for future predictive and personalized medicine.

Combining the strengths of the knowledge base of traditional systems of medicine with the dramatic power of combinatorial sciences and HTS will help in the generation of structure–activity libraries which will converge to form a real discovery engine that can result in newer, safer, cheaper and effective therapies.

The traditional systems of medicine in Asia (Ayurveda, TCM, SCM, Kampo) are considered great living traditions. They are all closely related to each other. For example, all are based on theories of constitution. All identify unique qualities of each individual, and state the necessity of developing personalized medicine in order to obtain optimal response to treatment. This is similar to the science of Pharmacogenomics, which tries to identify individual differences between patients connected to drug metabolism, efficacy and toxicity at the genomic level. Current research in 'Omics' is focusing on the polygenic approach using high throughput technology rather than the single gene approach.

Such research found a genetic basis for the classification of physical constitution in traditional medicine. "These observations are likely to have an impact on phenotype-genotype correlation, drug discovery, pharmacogenomics and personalized medicine." So, "Identifying genetic variations in Asia-based constitution may provide a newer approach to pharmacogenomics and help better understand the scientific classification basis of human population for better therapeutic benefits."

4. Current status: Promises and bottle necks

4.1 Appraisals or evidence for importance of Ayurveda

The evidence is what is required to prove an idea or concept or even a system. There exist plethora of evidence for scientific basis of Ayurveda (Mishra 2003; Patwardhan& Mashelkar 2009; Vaidya AB 2006) and one needs to adopt an unbiased neutral opinion to see the promising way forward for drug discovery with support of Ayurveda. Because ancient sciences are not limited to one religion or geographical area, they should be used for benefit of health care system in totality. The promising outputs are already available where Ayurveda has given many miracle drugs like Ashwagandha (*Withania somnifera*, Family: Solanaceae), Guggul (*Commiphora wightii*, F: Burseraceae), Shatavari (*Asparagus racemosus*, F: Asparagaceae), Brahmi(*Centella asiatica*, F: Mackinlayaceae), Neem (*Azadirachta indica*, F: Meliaceae), Turmeric (*Curcuma longa*, F: Zingiberaceae), Isabgul (*Plantago ovata*, F: Plantaginaceae) so on and so forth. These drugs can be used both in traditional forms as well as in form of standardized semipurified or purified phytopharmaceuticals. These plants or their parts are regulated differently in different countries. As per Ayurvedic system of medicine they are licensed as drugs and are in Clinical use in India. As these drugs are not fully standardised or as currently there is no globally accepted common regulations for herbals they can be considered as herbal supplement or functional food etc.

The research on preclinical, clinical, Phytochemical, Pharmacokinetics-Pharmacodynemics (PK-PD), safety pharmacology etc. for ayurvedic drugs and formulations are on surge and world needs to have more integrative and planned approach so as to leverage the benefit of this tie-up between ancient and contemporary sciences.

4.2 Possible bottle necks

As many concepts of Ayurveda are more of integrated nature it needs inputs from many branches of science. As for example personalized medicine concept is an integral part of Ayurveda and is based on "Prakriti" of an individual which affects the choice of medicine and the way the particular health condition is treated though Ayurveda. This paradigm is into its infancy in modern science where we are still trying to understand genetic variations and their links with diseases and physiology. One of the possible bottlenecks can be lack of scientific tools which help to understand the detailed concepts of Ayurveda.

Another bottle neck that is already under debate is "marker" based evaluation of herbs. Traditionally ayurvedic herbs are used in crude form (and not as isolated or purified compounds) and many a times in combination with other herbs or preparations and thus science behind chemistry of such complex mixtures is yet to be evolved. Even though Ayurveda has provided many promising leads in terms of isolated molecules it is different part of story where individual phytoconstituents are studied as drugs. Thus we need to differentiate between traditional ayurvedic drugs and modern form of phyto-constituent based drugs (Patwardhan& Mashelkar 2009).

5. Win-win situation for future of health care

To conclude this chapter we would like to elaborate various points where ancient science of Ayurveda and contemporary health care stream can gain from each other for far reaching benefits and newer directions of drug discovery and health.

Table No. 4 discusses benefits that can be gained by Ayurveda and contemporary science.

6. Disclaimer

Dr Kapil M Khambholja is currently affiliated to Novartis Healthcare Pvt. Ltd., India and was earlier affiliated to S K Patel College of Pharmacetuical Education and Research, Ganpat University, India as an Asst. Professor. The views expressed in this chapter are purely of author him self and in no manner reflects views or opinion from affiliating company or organisation.

	Benefits for Ayurveda	Benefits for drug discovery / health care sciences
Benefits in Chemistry domain	- Understanding of chemistry behind success of ayurvedic herbs. - Better understanding of chemical transformation during traditional manufacturing practices	- Availability of new leads based on SAR studies of phytoconstituents. - Herbo-mineral formulations mixed with plants provide unique combination for studying interaction between organic and inorganic constitutents.
Benefits in Process domain	- Ability to provide uniform and consistent products using analytical and standardisation techniques - Traditional manufacturing techniques can be improved using modern unit operation based techniques.	- Traditional ayurvedic manufacturing techniques involve unique type of processes which can form basis of improved unique processes of purification, separation, manufacturing etc.
Benefits in Life science domain	- better understanding of mechanisms of individual herbs using invitro techniques - better understanding of mechanisms of polyherbal formulations using in-vivo animal models - Understanding genetic basis of prakriti and tri-dosha based classification of humans	- Improved understanding of correlation between mind and body linked with quantum physics / chemistry - Newer approaches for maintaing health and /or treating diseased conditions. - Understanding of link between life style, environment and health

Table 4. Win-win situation for Ayurveda, contemporary drug discovery process and health care sciences

7. References

(2000). *General Guidelines for Methodologies on Research and Evaluation of Traditional Medicine.* Geneva: World Health Organisation.

Aggarwal S, Negi S, Jha P, Singh PK, Stobdan T, Pasha MA, Ghosh S, Agrawal A, Prasher B , Mukerji M (2010). EGLN1 involvement in high-altitude adaptation revealed through genetic analysis of extreme constitution types defined in Ayurveda. *Proc Natl Acad Sci U S A.* Vol.107,No., 44, 18961-18966.1091-6490 (Electronic) 0027-8424 (Linking),

Patwardhan B (2007). *Drug discovery and development: traditional medicine and ethnopharmacology.* New Delhi: New India Publishing Agency.

Patwardhan B, Joshi K, Arvind C (2005). Classification of Human Population Based on HLA Gene Polymorphism and the Concept of Prakriti in Ayurveda. *The Journal of Alternative and Complementary Medicine.* Vol.11,No., 2, 349-353,

Bhushan Patwardhan, Ashok Vaidya, Mukund Chorghade (2004). Ayurveda and natural products drug discovery. *Current Science.* Vol.86,No., 6, 789-799,

Chopra A, Saluja M, Tillu G, Venugopalan A, Sarmukaddam S, Raut AK, Bichile L, Narsimulu G, Handa R , Patwardhan B (2011). A Randomized Controlled Exploratory Evaluation of Standardized Ayurvedic Formulations in Symptomatic Osteoarthritis Knees: A Government of India NMITLI Project. *Evidence-based Complementary and Alternative Medicine.* Vol.2011,No.,

Gautam M, Saha S, Bani S, Kaul A, Mishra S, Patil D, Satti NK, Suri KA, Gairola S, Suresh K, Jadhav S, Qazi GN , Patwardhan B (2009). Immunomodulatory activity of Asparagus racemosus on systemic Th1/Th2 immunity: Implications for immunoadjuvant potential. *Journal of Ethnopharmacology.* Vol.121,No., 2, 241-247.0378-8741,

Ghodke Y, Joshi K , Patwardhan B (2009). Traditional Medicine to Modern Pharmacogenomics: Ayurveda Prakriti Type and CYP2C19 Gene Polymorphism Associated with the Metabolic Variability. *Evid Based Complement Alternat Med.*No.1741-4288 (Electronic) 1741-427X (Linking),

Gupta R, Gabrielsen B , Ferguson SM (2005). Nature's medicines: traditional knowledge and intellectual property management. Case studies from the National Institutes of Health (NIH), USA. *Curr Drug Discov Technol.* Vol.2,No., 4, 203-219.1570-1638 (Print) 1570-1638 (Linking),

Harvey AL (2008). Natural products in drug discovery. *Drug Discov Today.* Vol.13,No., 19-20, 894-901.1359-6446 (Print) 1359-6446 (Linking),

Joshi K, Hankey A , Patwardhan B (2007). Traditional Phytochemistry: Identification of Drug by ‘Taste&#x2019. *Evidence-based Complementary and Alternative Medicine.* Vol.4,No., 2, 145-148,

Levy S, Sutton G, Ng PC, Feuk L, Halpern AL, Walenz BP, Axelrod N, Huang J, Kirkness EF, Denisov G, Lin Y, MacDonald JR, Pang AWC, Shago M, Stockwell TB, Tsiamouri A, Bafna V, Bansal V, Kravitz SA, Busam DA, Beeson KY, McIntosh TC, Remington KA, Abril JF, Gill J, Borman J, Rogers Y-H, Frazier ME, Scherer SW, Strausberg RL , Venter JC (2007). The Diploid Genome Sequence of an Individual Human. *PLoS Biol.* Vol.5,No., 10, e254,

Mashelkar RA (2008). Second World Ayurveda Congress (Theme: Ayurveda for the Future) - Inaugural address: Part I. *Evidence-based Complementary and Alternative Medicine.* Vol.5,No., 2, 129-131.1741-427X,

Mishra L.(2003).*Scientific basis of Ayurvedic Therapies,* CRC Press, 0-8493-1366-X, New Yourk

Patwardhan B , Mashelkar RA (2009). Traditional medicine-inspired approaches to drug discovery: can Ayurveda show the way forward? *Drug Discov Today.* Vol.14,No., 15-16, 804-811.1878-5832 (Electronic)1359-6446 (Linking),

Prasher B, Negi S, Aggarwal S, Mandal AK, Sethi TP, Deshmukh SR, Purohit SG, Sengupta S, Khanna S, Mohammad F, Garg G, Brahmachari SK , Mukerji M (2008). Whole genome expression and biochemical correlates of extreme constitutional types defined in Ayurveda. *J Transl Med.* Vol.6,No., 48.1479-5876 (Electronic) 1479-5876 (Linking),

Puranik AS, Halade G, Kumar S, Mogre R, Apte K, Vaidya ADB , Patwardhan B (2011). Cassia auriculata: Aspects of Safety Pharmacology and Drug Interaction. *Evidence-based Complementary and Alternative Medicine.* Vol.2011,No.,

Sharma H , Chandola HM (2011). Prameha in Ayurveda: Correlation with Obesity, Metabolic Syndrome, and Diabetes Mellitus. Part 1â€"Etiology, Classification, and Pathogenesis. *The Journal of Alternative and Complementary Medicine.* Vol.17,No., 6, 491-496,

Sharma P (1995). *Charak Samhita.* Varanasi, India: Chaukambha Orientallia.

Steinberg KK, Gwinn M , Khoury MJ (2001). The Role of Genomics in Public Health and Disease Prevention. *JAMA: The Journal of the American Medical Association.* Vol.286,No., 13, 1635,

Sumantran VN, Kulkarni A, Chandwaskar R, Harsulkar A, Patwardhan B, Chopra A , Wagh UV (2008). Chondroprotective Potential of Fruit Extracts of Phyllanthus emblica in Osteoarthritis. *Evidence-based Complementary and Alternative Medicine.* Vol.5,No., 3, 329-335,

Tripathi J, Reddy KRC, Gupta S , Dubey S (2010). A comparative clinical trial on the role of *Panchakarma therapy* and *Unmada Gajankusha Rasa* in the cases of major depressive disorder vis-à-vis *kaphaja Unmada. AYU (An international quarterly journal of research in Ayurveda).* Vol.31,No., 2, 205-209,

Vaidya AB RA (2006). Evidences based Ayurveda Sorting fact from fantasy. In *Ayurveda and its Scientific Aspects - Opportunities for Globalisation).* New Delhi: Department of AYUSH and CSIR, pp. 1-30.

4

Novel Oncology Drug Development Strategies in the Era of Personalised Medicine

C.R. Lemech[1,2], R.S. Kristeleit[2] and H.T. Arkenau[1,2]

[1]Sarah Cannon Research UK, London

[2]Cancer Institute, University College London

UK

1. Introduction

In this era of personalised medicine, the focus of oncology drug development is shifting from classic chemotherapeutic drugs to rationally designed molecularly targeted agents (MTAs). This development has been accelerated by improved understanding of the key features of human tumour biology which have emerged over the last decade. A seminal paper by Hanahan and Weinberg (2000) proposed six vital elements for tumour formation, survival and progression. The six 'Hallmarks of Cancer' were sustained proliferative signalling, evasion of growth suppressors, resistance to cell death, replicative immortality, angiogenesis and activation of invasion and metastasis. Hanahan and Weinberg updated their findings in 2011 with further evidence describing the complexity of these hallmarks and the addition of further hallmarks, including modification of energy metabolism to fuel cell growth and evasion of immunosurveillance. The tumour micro-environment is also a critical factor in the regulation of tumour growth and progression, with multiple stromal cell types creating a succession of supportive tumour micro-environments enabling invasion of normal tissue and subsequent metastasis.

Recent successes have utilised these advances in understanding to create a strong biologic rationale for drug development, primarily focusing on targets of a single 'Hallmark'.

However, a number of challenges remain, not only in understanding the complex molecular pathways and networks, their interaction and mechanisms of resistance, but also in the drug development process through early incorporation of biomarkers to create rational drug development strategies. Challenges also lie in defining robust criteria to appropriately select patients for novel therapies. Effective trial design with integration of patient enrichment strategies is paramount to streamline drug development and deliver timely information to guide progress of drugs along the pipeline. The application of new technologies and novel strategies that address these problems will be discussed in detail in this chapter.

2. From hypothesis to proof of concept

Historically, the emphasis for drug development has focused on evidence-based medicine in large trials of unselected patient populations, with the benchmark endpoint for new drugs being overall survival or other intermediate endpoints. This 'one size fits all' paradigm did not always take into account intra- and interpatient tumour heterogeneity commonly leading to large scale failure rates of multinational phase-III trials.

Incorporating measures of pathway activity and tumour efficacy into early phase trials may help avoid failure in later phases of drug development. Early validation of pharmacodynamic assays to measure target blockade and assess optimal dose range and dosing schedule is essential. Establishing 'proof-of-concept' can then correlate anti-tumour activity in a selected patient population with validated predictive and intermediate endpoint biomarkers (De Bono & Ashworth., 2010).

For example, in patients with non-small cell lung cancer (NSCLC), correlation of epidermal growth factor receptor (EGFR) mutations with response to the EGFR inhibitors, gefitinib or erlotinib, occurred only after a number of negative trials. Although phase-II data in the second-line setting in patients with NSCLC was encouraging, when taken to a phase-III trial in an unselected group of patients with refractory disease, gefitinib failed to show a benefit in either overall survival or time-to-treatment failure when compared to placebo (Thatcher et al., 2005). In this context, it was only that retrospective analyses could help identify a sub-population benefiting from treatment including being a female, never-smoker and of Asian origin. Similarly, erlotinib demonstrated progression-free and overall survival benefits both in the second-line setting and as maintenance therapy in patients with stable disease after first-line chemotherapy (Cappuzzo et al., 2010; Shepherd et al., 2005). However, the incremental benefits in these unselected patient populations were small, measured in weeks for progression-free survival and 1-2 months for overall survival. Ultimately it was the selection of patients based on EGFR mutation status that demonstrated a marked improvement in response rates and survival in phase-III trials comparing chemotherapy and gefitinib (Fukuoka et al., 2011), as well as chemotherapy and erlotinib in the first-line setting (Rosell et al., 2011).

We have witnessed similar studies in patients with advanced colorectal cancer (ACRC) treated with the monoclonal antibody cetuximab. Initially, treatment with cetuximab was conducted in patients with EGFR over-expression, assessed by immunohistochemistry (IHC) on formalin-fixed paraffin-embedded (FFPE) tumour specimens (Cunningham et al., 2004). It was only later that the importance of Kirsten rat sarcoma-2 virus oncogene (KRAS) mutation was demonstrated; and this, in combination with an increased understanding of the complex EGFR downstream signalling cascade were the first steps in identifying a predictive biomarker for EGFR directed therapies in patients with ACRC. Several studies identified that patients with KRAS mutation did not respond to EGFR directed therapies, whereas patients who had wildtype (wt) KRAS tumours had response rates of over 50% (Lievre et al., 2006; Karapetis et al., 2008). More recently, it has been demonstrated that in fact, not all KRAS mutations are created equal. Although the presence of the majority of KRAS mutations precludes response to the EGFR inhibitors in ACRC, other KRAS mutations, particularly in codon 13, may predict a response similar to that demonstrated in wt KRAS tumours (De Roock et al., 2010).

These are just a few examples that demonstrate how the improved understanding of tumour biology supports a hypothesis-driven approach to the discovery of compounds to potentially generate more selective inhibition of key signalling proteins, pathways and networks. In this context, one of the most challenging tasks is the identification of the right target and more importantly whether this target is 'druggable'. For example, although we know that RAS mutations are an early component of tumorigenesis and are identified in approximately 30% of human cancers, attempts to target RAS have been unsuccessful to date as complex molecular structures constrain binding to the active site or pocket (Gysin et al., 2011). In contrast, selective inhibition of the v-raf murine sarcoma viral oncogene homologue B1 (BRAF) in patients with BRAF V600 mutant melanoma is associated with a dramatic improvement in response rates and survival. The strong biologic rationale of this approach was established through identification of the importance of the mitogen-activated protein kinase (MAPK) pathway in this disease and will be discussed at a later point in this chapter.

3. Biomarker development

Predictive and prognostic biomarkers are increasingly important in tailoring treatment decisions for individual patients. These markers are objectively measured to evaluate pathological processes or pharmacological responses to a therapeutic intervention, and can be any kind of molecule, substance, or genetic marker which is traceable (Atkinson et al., 2001). Predictive biomarkers provide information on response to a treatment, whereas prognostic biomarkers give information about outcome independent of the treatment effect. Historically, biomarkers have often been developed in retrospective analyses and were only in some cases prospectively applied. The retrospective approach was often criticised for being slow and difficult in practice, as well as raising concerns regarding heterogenous sample collection and validity. There are increasing efforts to incorporate new biomarker strategies into the earliest stages of clinical trial design, whether these are mutational analyses, clinical, or imaging measures, so that information can be gathered early and continually revisited during and after trial completion to inform the clinical development process.

As witnessed with a number of targeted agents, such as trastuzumab in human epidermal growth factor receptor-2 (HER2) positive breast cancer, the prospective analysis of HER2 as a predictive biomarker in clinical trials resulted in higher response rates and increased survival in this selected patient population, both in the metastatic and adjuvant setting (Slamon et al., 2001; Romond et al., 2005). This selective approach not only led to better outcomes for this subgroup, but ultimately to shorter and streamlined regulatory approval timelines. The use of trastuzumab in an unselected breast cancer population would undoubtedly have masked its true efficacy and potentially curtailed its development.

Importantly this selective biomarker approach became a good example of what challenges researchers are facing when developing accurate, functional and standardised biomarker assays.

HER2 gene amplification was first observed to be a potential biomarker in breast cancer when its presence in 25% of axillary lymph-node positive breast cancers was correlated with worse prognosis (Slamon et al., 1987). Additional studies confirmed that HER2 protein over-expression was also a poor prognostic marker in breast cancer, correlating with decreased relapse-free and overall survival (Ravdin et al., 1995). The trastuzumab clinical trials were initially designed using HER2 over-expression measured by IHC with a centralised sponsor developed assay, which was particularly important as there was no standardised assay at that time. As the testing of HER2 was expanded from central to local laboratories, with incorporation of fluorescence in-situ hybridisation (FISH) in addition to IHC, there were concerns about the correlation and regulation of such assays.

Although the results of the five adjuvant trastuzumab trials in HER2 positive early stage breast cancer clearly showed a significant clinical benefit in both progression-free and overall survival, the testing algorithms for HER2 were not consistent across these trials. HER2 testing included either IHC supported by FISH testing for intermediate IHC result (IHC2+) or reliance on FISH testing alone to assess gene amplification ratios. Concern was generated at the lack of accuracy and validation of HER2 testing in some instances as several assays were in use, including both validated assays, but also so called "home brew" assays developed in local pathology laboratories. Sub-studies from two of the adjuvant trials demonstrated that approximately 20% of HER2 assays performed at the primary treatment site were incorrect compared to re-evaluation in a high volume, central laboratory (Paik et al., 2002; Roche et al., 2002). Furthermore, the sensitivity of IHC itself was of concern. For example, one study demonstrated that commercially available US Food and Drug Administration (FDA) approved IHC methods were significantly less accurate than FISH at correctly characterising tumours with known HER2 status. Depending on the IHC method and use of HER2 antibody, correlation with FISH positivity ranged between 67-83%, with greater susceptibility to inter-observer variation (Bartlett et al., 2001).

Clearly in the case of IHC testing, several contributing factors may further impact on sensitivity and specificity including initial sample processing, time to and type of fixation, analytic variables of assay validation, equipment calibration, use of standardised laboratory procedures, training of staff, test reagents, use of standardised control materials and use of automated laboratory methods.

Slamon et al. (1989) demonstrated that a proportion of breast cancers known to have gene amplification and over-expression of HER2, in fact lose membrane staining after paraffin embedding and are negative on IHC assessment. Loss of antigenicity resulting in a potential false negative IHC can be affected by poor standardisation of fixative methods.

To overcome this lack of concordance in HER2 testing, which can so markedly impact on patients' prognosis and survival, an American Society of Clinical Oncology (ASCO) panel developed guidelines to improve the accuracy of HER2 testing (Wolff et al., 2007). These recommendations covered over 30 aspects of testing and requirements including the HER2 testing algorithm, optimal FISH and IHC testing and interpretation, tissue handling, internal validation and quality assurance procedures, optimal external proficiency, laboratory accreditation and regulatory requirements, statistical requirements for assay validation and international external quality assessment initiatives. Despite these guidelines, there were concerns that IHC assessment still lacked sufficient sensitivity to be used alone to decide on HER2 status (Carlson., 2008) though this remains the standard initial assessment in most laboratories.

In 2010, the addition of trastuzumab to first-line chemotherapy in HER2 positive advanced gastric cancer demonstrated a survival benefit (Bang et al., 2010). Similar to breast cancer, approximately 20-30% of gastric and gastro-oesophageal junction (GOJ) cancers show HER2 over-expression, but the testing criteria in gastric specimens differs significantly (Albarello et al., 2011). This is related to the increased frequency of heterogeneity of HER2 positivity in gastric cancer compared with breast cancer, as well as variations in membrane staining and the number of stained cells necessary to diagnose a positive case. In addition there is also less stringent correlation between HER2 amplification and protein over-expression with more than 20% of cases carrying HER2 amplification, often of low level, without HER2 expression. Clinically in this group of patients, there is no apparent benefit from adding trastuzumab to chemotherapy (Bang et al., 2010). Similarly, Hofmann et al. (2008a) demonstrated concordance between FISH and IHC of 93%, with 7% of specimens demonstrating FISH positivity with negative or equivocal IHC staining.

Discordant findings have also been demonstrated with HER2 testing on surgical specimens compared to biopsy alone, with more than 10% of cases showing discrepant results (Yano et al., 2006). As a result, if only gastric or GOJ cancer biopsy samples are available for HER2 testing, current guidelines recommend sampling of at least 6 different areas of the tumour for HER2 analysis. New IHC scoring criteria have also been developed for gastric and GOJ cancers and were validated by Hofmann et al. (2008b), further demonstrating that the analysis of HER2 based on the breast cancer guidelines may lead to false negative reporting in gastric cancer specimens.

This example demonstrates that although an assay may have progressed through thorough validation and review processes in one cancer sub-type, its use cannot be assumed for other malignancies and re-validation needs to be incorporated into early phase trials, particularly when the drug is readily available and may otherwise rapidly proceed to clinical practice. Furthermore, when several IHC assays exist, it is of the utmost importance that laboratories validate their internal IHC and FISH procedures according to international guidelines.

In this context it is paramount that biomarker development is orchestrated collaboratively in large multi-institutional networks. The integration of biomarkers early in drug development and correlation with clinical observations can generate early signals of unexpected efficacy or resistance that can then be used to change the direction of development of a particular drug and enhance outcomes.

Furthermore new health information technologies (HIT) are a pivotal part of biomarker development and need to be linked into routine practice to support the large-scale information of tumour biology and clinical data. The use of HIT will also support the integration of a variety of data sets including gene expression profiles, metabolic, immunohistochemical profiles and clinical outcome data. The development of next generation sequencing, functional genomic screening and transcriptional analysis offers detailed insight not only into DNA sequence, but also into mRNA profiles, protein structure and metabolic pathways. The enormity of the information that is available needs parallel information technologies to interpret and link these findings to their regulated networks. The ultimate application of these technologies involves the modelling of interacting pathways to make phenotypic predictions and develop complete system models to advance personalised drug development. The incorporation of molecular biology and information technology can thus maximise the interpretation, application and targeting of these complex oncological systems. In this context, bioinformatics has evolved to combine sequence matching and pattern discovery with modelling of dynamic biological systems to enhance the drug discovery process.

4. Developments of new rationally designed targeted therapies

Several recent phase-I trials of molecularly targeted agents have demonstrated remarkable progress when patients were selected based on their molecular profile and subsequently treated with an agent directed against this specific target.

The shift from 'one size fits all' to molecularly defined subpopulations has been particularly successful in the treatment of patients with advanced BRAF mutant cutaneous melanoma. Two pivotal phase-I trials, showed encouraging response rates and improved survival rates with the selective BRAF inhibitors, vemurafenib (PLX4032) and GSK 2118436, in a disease notoriously resistant to standard chemotherapies. Another trial in patients with NSCLC who were carriers of the EML4-ALK fusion protein showed remarkable response rates with the new ALK inhibitor, crizotinib. The successful development of such agents is of course complex but can be simplistically considered as having three key components: the right target (strong biologic rationale, druggable), the right drug (selective, right formulation, tolerable side-effect profile) and the right biomarker (reproducible, validated) (Figure 1). This paradigm can be further evidenced by the success of imatinib and CAL-101 in haematological malignancies and reflects the limitations that have impacted on the use of other agents, such as sorafenib in melanoma or bevacizumab in breast and other malignancies.

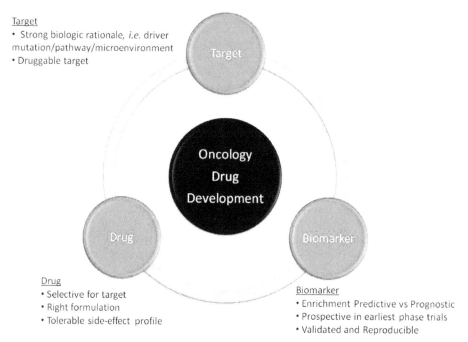

Fig. 1. Key Components of Oncology Drug Development

Sorafenib is an oral multikinase inhibitor of vascular endothelial growth factor receptor (VEGFR), platelet derived growth factor receptor (PDGFR)-β and Raf-1 (Wilhelm et al., 2006). Although it was initially developed as a RAF inhibitor, sorafenib showed only moderate IC50s for all three RAF isoforms and also had inhibitory effects on several other receptor tyrosine kinases including VEGFR2, VEGFR3, PDGFRβ, cKIT and FLT3. Sorafenib has demonstrated significant improvements both in clinical benefit rate and survival in renal cell carcinoma (RCC) and hepatocellular carcinoma (HCC) (Escudier et al., 2005; Llovet et al., 2008). Correlative markers were incorporated into these trials including phosphorylated ERK (pERK) immunostaining and soluble c-KIT, VEGFR2, VEGFR3 and VEGF levels. As yet however, there is no validated biomarker to predict the target patient population.

Despite a good biologic rationale to support its use in melanoma and promising early phase trials, sorafenib failed to show a clinical benefit in phase II-III trials (Eisen et al., 2006; Hauschild et al., 2009). Unlike the early phase trials for the selective BRAF inhibitors, patients were not selected for BRAF mutations, one of the key drivers in cutaneous melanoma, nor were the pharmacodynamic markers from the early phase trials translated into the design of the phase-III trials. The failure of this drug development programme in melanoma could have been mitigated if phase-II data had been critically reviewed and early 'go or no-go' decisions had been incorporated in the decision making process for the phase-III trials.

Similarly, the development of bevacizumab as a drug targeting the 'angiogenic switch' and tumour-associated neo-vasculature met with much anticipation (Hanahan & Folkman, 1996). Bevacizumab is a humanised monoclonal antibody targeting VEGF-A and its binding to VEGFR2. There was early pre-clinical evidence that it not only inhibited the formation of new blood vessels, but also caused regression of existing micro-vessels and stabilised the mature vasculature to improve drug delivery. Significant clinical benefit Has been demonstrated with bevacizumab in combination with chemotherapy in advanced colorectal cancer but despite promising data regarding potential clinical, biochemical and radiological parameters, a predictive biomarker remains elusive (Hurwitz et al., 2004; Jubb & Harris, 2010). Although bevacizumab is now approved in several disease entities, the broad use in many tumour types remains controversial, bearing in mind its associated cost and toxicity. In this context, the lack of proven and validated biomarkers to predict the patient population most likely to benefit is often criticised and in part may have contributed to the withdrawal by the FDA of its approval in metastatic breast cancer.

On the contrary, the development of selective BRAF inhibitors for BRAF V600 mutation positive advanced cutaneous melanoma commenced with a strong biologic rationale and its success was facilitated by the validation of an associated predictive biomarker (Figure 2). Aberrant activation of the MAPK pathway has been demonstrated in over 80% of primary melanomas, due to abnormalities at various levels' along the RAS-RAF-MEK-ERK pathway with subsequent acceleration of cell growth, proliferation and differentiation (Platz et al., 2008). BRAF mutations are among the most studied, occurring in 36-59% of primary melanomas (Houben et al., 2004; Jakob et al., 2011; Long et al., 2011) and 42-66% of metastatic melanomas and have been characterised as oncogenic mutations (Davies et al., 2002; Karasarides et al., 2004). Early phase trials with the selective BRAF inhibitors, vemurafenib (PLX4032) and GSK 2118436, have demonstrated response rates far higher than standard chemotherapy with impressive improvements in survival (Chapman et al., 2011; Flaherty et al., 2010; Kefford et al., 2010; Ribas et al., 2011.). Thus, the identification of 'the right target', the BRAF mutation, lent itself to the development of 'the right drug', the selective BRAF inhibitors, whose efficacy could be predicted by 'the right biomarker', presence of a BRAF mutation.

Activating mutations or translocations of the anaplastic lymphoma kinase gene (ALK) have been identified in several types of cancer, with the EML4-ALK fusion gene evident in 2-7% of all NSCLC. EML4-ALK is an aberrant fusion gene that encodes a cytoplasmic chimeric protein with constitutive kinase activity. It is more prevalent in patients who are never or light smokers and in patients with adenocarcinoma histology. Crizotinib is a selective inhibitor of the ALK and MET tyrosine kinases and has shown unprecedented response rates and clinical benefit in a phase-I trial of heavily pretreated patients with advanced NSCLC harbouring ALK rearrangement (Kwak et al., 2010). The study incorporated molecular analysis of tumour samples with prospective tumour genotyping, including analysis via FISH, IHC and reverse-transcriptase-polymerase-chain-reaction (RT-PCR). FISH positivity for ALK rearrangement strongly correlated with aberrant expression of the ALK protein on IHC and many patients, though not all, also had positive results for EML4-ALK on the RT-PCR assay. The use of prospective tumour genotyping not only potentiated the development of diagnostic approaches for these patients but has also streamlined rapid drug development for crizotinib. Remarkably, there were only three years between target identification, initiation of the phase-I trial and enrolment on the phase-III registration trial and stands in contrast to more than ten years from the initial unsuccessful trials of EGFR inhibitors in non-genotyped unselected patients to the phase–III trials that demonstrated benefit of EGFR inhibitors in EGFR-mutant tumours (Kwak et al., 2010). Again, there is strong supporting evidence for *'the right target'* and *'the right drug'* in this setting, whilst development of *'the right biomarker'* has been incorporated into the phase-I trials to assist in overcoming the many complexities inherent with new assay validation.

1. Development of a strong biologic rationale
Mutations along the MAPK pathway present in up to 80% of metastatic melanomas
In vitro evidence with vemurafenib (PLX4032) and GSK 2118436 of selective inhibition of BRAF V600E and impaired tumour growth in mouse models
2. Biomarkers for early phase trials
Prognostic Biomarker: BRAF aberrations
Predictive Biomarker: BRAF V600E aberrations (and V600K with GSK118436)
Pharmacodynamic Biomarkers: pMEK and pERK
3. Confirmation of a clinical response
Phase 1/2 trials (vemurafenib): RR 50-80%; PFS >7m
Phase 1/2 trials (GSK 2118436): RR 60%; PFS 8.3m
Phase 3 trial (vemurafenib vs dacarbazine): RR 48% v 5%; PFS 5.3m v 1.6m OS at 6m 84% v 64%
4. Dissecting the Mechanisms of Resistance
Longitudinal biopsies pre-treatment, on treatment and on progression
On-target effect demonstrated by suppression of pMEK and pERK, and decreased staining of proliferative markers on IHC (cyclin D1 and Ki67)
Resistance possible through alternate signalling in MAPK pathway or via bypass pathway signalling
Vemurafenib
Some tumours demonstrate increased pMEK/pERK on progression with reactivation of MAPK pathway
Evidence of NRAS and MEK mutations which mediate signalling via the MAPK pathway
Evidence of PTEN loss and increase pAkt demonstrates activation of PI3K-AKT-mTOR pathway
GSK 2118436
Abnormal PTEN associated with shorter PFS and loss of inhibition of the PI3K-AKT pathway
CDKN2A and KIT deletion associated with shorter PFS

MAPK: mitogen-activated protein kinase; IHC: immunohistochemistry;
BRAF: v-raf murine sarcoma viral oncogene homologue B1;
pMEK: phosphorylated MEK; pERK: phosphorylated ERK; pAKT: phosphorylated AKT; RR: response rate; PFS: progression-free survival, OS: overall survival;
PI3K: phosphatidylinositol 3-kinase; mTOR: mammalian target of rapamycin

Fig. 2. Selective BRAF Inhibitors for BRAF mutant Metastatic Melanoma

In haematological malignancies, the development of the phosphatidylinositol 3-kinase (PI3K) inhibitor, CAL-101, has shown encouraging results in advanced non-hodgkins lymphoma (NHL), mantle cell lymphoma and chronic lymphocytic leukaemia (CLL) (Herman et al., 2010). CAL-101 is a selective inhibitor of the PI3K p110 δ isoform that is primarily expressed on cells of haematopoietic origin and has a key role in B cell maturation and function. Through inhibition of PI3K signalling, CAL-101 can induce apoptosis of primary CLL and acute myelogenous leukaemia (AML) cells and a range of other leukaemia and lymphoma cell lines (Lannutti et al., 2010). In phase–I studies, CAL-101 has demonstrated durable clinical responses in a number of haematological malignancies, including NHL (Flinn et al., 2009). Reduction in phosphorylated AKT (pAKT) as a marker of PI3K activation provides *'proof-of-mechanism'* for this agent and later phase trials are underway in B cell malignancies with markers along the PI3Kδ pathway acting as predictive biomarkers.

These recent *'proof-of-concept'* studies were the first of their kind where molecular profiles were used for selection of *'new in class'* compounds and demonstrate that when patients are appropriately selected, convincing benefit can be realised in the earliest of trials, setting the stage for rapid drug approval. This phase-I experience has convinced investigators that tumour profiling and patient selection will become a routine part of cancer drug development.

5. Challenges in drug development

5.1 Mechanisms of resistance

Despite the advances in parallel drug and biomarker development in early clinical trials, one of the major challenges remaining is the understanding of mechanisms that cause primary and acquired or secondary resistance. Primary resistance is characterised by lack of efficacy of an agent from treatment initiation, whereas acquired resistance develops after an initial response of some degree over a period of time.

As evidenced by all currently approved molecularly targeted agents, initial treatment may yield response rates far higher than standard chemotherapy with impressive disease control, but inevitably resistance and tumour progression develops. Importantly, understanding the mechanisms of resistance can lead to rationally designed drug combinations incorporating targeted agents, antibodies, or cytotoxics. This approach should include continuous analysis of tumour material via biopsies on disease progression or surrogate markers such as circulating tumour cells (CTCs) or circulating free DNA (cfDNA). In this context, cancer treatment could follow strategies as witnessed by the treatment of tuberculosis with quadruple combination regimens or human immunodeficiency virus (HIV) with highly active antiretroviral therapy (HAART). In a similar way, cancer drugs will be used in parallel or sequentially to block different driver pathways and networks simultaneously.

Although there are a number of mechanisms of resistance that are particular to molecularly targeted agents and are intrinsic to the pathway they inhibit, there are other mechanisms that are common to both cytotoxic chemotherapy and molecularly targeted agents falling into three main categories: decreased uptake, such as occurs with water-soluble drugs like the folate antagonists; impaired capacity of cytoxic drugs to induce cell kill via a combination of altered cell cycle checkpoints, increased or altered drug targets, repair of DNA damage and inhibition of apoptosis; or increased drug efflux (Gottesman et al., 2002; Szakacs et al., 2006).

The presence of efflux pumps is one of the best described mechanisms of resistance and is thought to be common to both cytotoxic chemotherapy and the molecularly targeted agents. P-glycoprotein (P-gp), otherwise known as the multidrug transporter, is an energy dependent efflux pump that has been identified as a major mechanism of multidrug resistance (MDR) in cultured cancer cells. It is the product of the MDR1 gene in humans and is one member of a large family of ATP-dependent transporters known as the ATP-binding cassette (ABC family). P-gp is widely expressed in many human cancers including cancers of the gastrointestinal tract, hematopoietic system, genitourinary system and childhood cancers. P-gp can detect and bind a large variety of hydrophobic natural-product drugs as they enter the plasma membrane including chemotherapeutic agents such as doxorubicin, vinblastine and paclitaxel, as well as anti-arrhythmics, antihistamines and the HIV protease inhibitors (Robert., 1999). Increased drug efflux was initially thought to be a significant mechanism of resistance for the tyrosine kinase inhibitor imatinib in patients with CML (Mahon et al., 2003). However, it is not fully understood how much impact this resistance mechanism has on molecularly targeted drugs as a prime source of resistance.

Another relevant mechanism of resistance that has been illustrated in a number of cancers involves the disruption of interacting proteins and receptors on the plasma membrane level impacting on receptor binding and subsequent drug efficacy. For example, EGFR is a membrane-bound receptor whose signalling involves a complex pathway of ligand binding, receptor homo- and heterodimerisation with ERBB2 and other family members, followed by internalisation and recycling of the ligand-bound receptor. Significant EGF-dependent signalling may occur during the process of internalisation and alterations in EGFR trafficking have been linked to cellular responses (Wiley et al., 2003). Analysis of EGFR trafficking in resistant lung cancer cell lines demonstrated increased internalisation of EGFR compared to parental drug-sensitive cells, which interestingly could be overcome by the action of irreversible EGFR inhibitors (Kwak et al., 2005). Similarly in breast cancer, one of the proposed mechanisms of resistance to trastuzumab involves membrane-associated glycoprotein mucin-4 (MUC4) which may block the inhibitory actions of trastuzumab by directly binding with HER2 and preventing interaction between the drug and the molecular target (Nagy et al., 2005).

Primary or secondary mutations and aberrations at the level, up- or downstream of the target are also frequently studied mechanisms of resistance to the molecularly targeted agents. For example, primary resistance to the EGFR targeted agents, gefitinib and erlotinib, has been associated with the presence of a KRAS mutation in 20-30% of NSCLC patients, or via an insertion mutation in exon 20 of EGFR, which represents fewer than 5% of all known mutations in the EGFR gene (Hammerman et al., 2009). Secondary resistance to the EGFR inhibitors after an initial response is mediated by the T790M mutation in 50-59% of patients, characterised by the substitution of methionine for threonine at position 790 (T790M) in EGFR (Pao et al., 2005). In this case, biological understanding of primary and secondary resistance allows for development of rationally designed drugs. Pre-clinical evidence demonstrated that an irreversible inhibitor of EGFR, such as neratinib (HKI-272), could overcome resistance induced by T790M-mutant EGFR and such agents are currently in clinical development (Kobayashi et al., 2005; Kwak et al., 2005).

Recent advances in the treatment of melanoma have further assisted in the understanding of the complexity of resistance mechanisms. For example although secondary BRAF mutations have not been identified as a cause of BRAF inhibitor resistance, mutations elsewhere along the MAPK pathway have been implicated, including secondary NRAS and MEK mutations.

MEK mutations have been demonstrated to cause reactivation of ERK signalling despite BRAF or MEK inhibition both in vitro and in vivo (Corcoran et al., 2011; Emery et al., 2009; Wagle et al., 2011). Similarly NRAS mutations, such as the NRAS Q61K mutation, have been demonstrated in BRAF mutant melanoma cell lines resistant to vemurafenib, and in a nodal biopsy from a patient who progressed after an initial response on treatment (Nazarian et al., 2010). The presence of an NRAS mutation can result in persistently elevated pMEK and pERK levels despite BRAF inhibition and is thought to signal through RAS and subsequently through RAF isoforms other then BRAF (Nazarian et al., 2010).

Signalling via the CRAF isoform is also a significant mechanism of resistance, with increased CRAF activity and a switch from BRAF to CRAF dependency demonstrated in BRAF mutant melanoma cell lines that are resistant to RAF inhibition (Montagut et al., 2008). Importantly, sensitivity to MEK inhibition was maintained in these cell lines, supporting further novel drug combinations, such as a non-selective RAF inhibitor or selective CRAF inhibitor with a MEK or BRAF inhibitor to overcome this mechanism of resistance.

Amplification of the mutant BRAF allele has also been implicated in resistance via increased pMEK and subsequently pERK signalling, though the evidence for this lies in studies of BRAF mutant colorectal cancer cell lines. In three such cell lines, BRAF amplification was demonstrated as a mechanism of acquired resistance to MEK inhibitors with cross-resistance to BRAF inhibitors, although to a lesser degree (Corcoran et al., 2010; Little et al., 2011). Preclinical studies showed that increased concentrations of RAF or MEK inhibitors, as well as the combination of the two agents, could suppress ERK phosphorylation and downstream signalling (Corcoran et al., 2010).

Changes in signalling upstream of a target pathway as well as bypass signalling along alternate pathways have also been demonstrated as mechanisms of resistance (Figure 3). In this context the insulin-like growth factor 1 receptor (IGF1R) which signals upstream of the PI3K-AKT-mTOR and MAPK pathways has been found to contribute to resistance in a number of malignancies. For example, activity of trastuzumab was impaired in breast cancer cells that over-expressed both HER2 and IGF1R, but its activity could be restored when IGF1R activation was blocked (Lu et al., 2001). Moreover, in vitro models have demonstrated that IGF1R physically interacts with and induces phosphorylation of HER2 in trastuzumab-resistant cells, but not in trastuzumab-sensitive cells, with subsequent increased signalling through the PI3K-AKT-mTOR and MAPK pathways. Again, inhibition of IGF1R signalling either by antibody blockade or tyrosine kinase inhibition restored trastuzumab sensitivity, demonstrating another potential therapeutic mechanism to overcome secondary resistance to trastuzumab. Similar findings were also evident in BRAF V600E melanoma cell lines resistant to BRAF inhibition, providing early evidence for the combination of IGF1R and MEK inhibition in this setting. (Villanueva et al., 2010).

A number of other preclinical studies have also demonstrated aberrant activation of the PI3K-AKT pathway at other levels that contributes to both primary and secondary resistance in BRAF mutant cell lines (Jiang et al., 2011; Shao et al., 2010). Just as the combination of IGF1R inhibition with MEK inhibition is being investigated to overcome resistance mediated along the IGF1R and MAPK pathways, there may be a biologic rationale for the combination of PI3K and MEK inhibitors (Jiang et al., 2010). In such cases, phosphorylated AKT may act as a marker of activity of the PI3K-AKT-mTOR pathway and thus, may be used as a biomarker to select when the combination of PI3K inhibitors and BRAF/MEK inhibitors is appropriate to block both the PI3K and MAPK pathways respectively.

PTEN loss (PTEN-) and subsequent lack of inhibition on the PI3K-AKT-mTOR pathway has also been demonstrated to confer resistance to BRAF inhibition. Paraiso et al. (2011) showed that in cell lines with PTEN loss compared to cell lines with normal PTEN, BRAF inhibition with vemurafenib was associated with increased AKT signalling and decreased apoptosis. Dual treatment of PTEN- cell lines with both vemurafenib and a PI3K inhibitor could then restore increased levels of apoptosis (Paraiso et al., 2011).

Exemplified by preclinical and clinical examples in melanoma, signalling via the PI3K-AKT-mTOR pathway mediates an important MAPK-pathway independent mechanism of resistance in a variety of cancers and demonstrates a complex crosstalk between these pathways (Corcoran et al., 2011). Measurement of phosphorylated ERK and phosphorylated AKT to determine pathway activity may therefore help to guide therapeutic choices and combinations of selective BRAF, MEK or PI3K/AKT inhibitors. Thus, knowledge of secondary resistance mechanisms will increasingly influence decision making processes for further drug development and rational drug combinations.

Although mechanisms of secondary resistance are well described for several new targeted agents, challenges remain, particularly with anti-angiogenic or multitargeted agents such as bevacizumab, sunitinib and sorafenib. The complexity of resistance mechanisms to anti-angiogenic therapy reflects the difficulty in developing anti-angiogenic agents in parallel with corresponding biomarkers.

So far, two main resistance mechanisms for anti-angiogenic agents have been proposed: firstly, evasive resistance with adaptation to circumvent specific angiogenic blockade, and secondly, intrinsic or pre-existing indifference (Bergers & Hanahan., 2008). Evasion of anti-angiogenic therapy may occur via up-regulation of alternative pro-angiogenic signalling circuits or via a number of alterations in the micro-environment, including recruitment of vascular progenitor cells and pro-angiogenic monocytes from the bone marrow, increased and tight pericyte coverage protecting tumour blood vessels and increased capacity for invasion without angiogenesis.

Alternate pro-angiogenic signals that have been implicated in preclinical studies include fibroblast growth factor (FGF)-1 and -2, ephrin A1 and A2 and angiopoietin-1. To establish the significance of these up-regulated genes, preclinical studies used the combination of FGF signalling suppression with VEGFR inhibitors and demonstrated that the combination of these agents attenuated re-vascularisation and slowed tumour growth (Casanovas et al., 2005). These findings were also seen clinically in patients with glioblastoma treated with the VEGFR inhibitor cediranib (Batchelor et al., 2007). After initial response, peripheral blood levels of FGF2 increased when patients progressed, suggesting that signalling through FGF assists in restoring angiogenesis. Elevated levels of pro-angiogenic factors such as VEGF and placental growth factor (PGF) have been previously proposed as predictive biomarkers for tumour response (Bocci et al., 2004). However there is also evidence that the expression of pro-angiogenic growth factors such as FGF, PDGF and others increase in advanced stages of metastatic breast cancer, resulting in alternate pathway signalling (Relf et al., 1997). Thus, there is uncertainty regarding the significance of these factors; whether the presence of pro-angiogenic factors in peripheral blood are in fact markers of response or resistance, or neither. Understanding the complex regulatory networks, the interaction of pro- and anti-angiogenic factors and contributing components of the micro-environment, illustrates the difficulties to-date in target and biomarker development, as well as the potential mechanisms by which anti-angiogenic therapy can be optimised.

Malignancy and Drug	Target	Biomarker	Mechanisms of Resistance Under investigation
Breast cancer			
Tamoxifen	Estrogen receptor	ER/PR status on IHC	Loss of ER expression Epigenetic changes in ER gene Increased drug metabolism ER/HER2 cross-talk PI3K-AKT pathway activation Alterations in co-regulatory proteins (Ring et al., 2004)
Trastuzumab	HER2 receptor	HER2 expression on IHC and/or FISH	MUC4 binding to HER2 (Nagy et al.; 2005) HER2 & IGF1R crosstalk (Lu et al., 2001) PI3K-AKT pathway signalling and PTEN loss
Bevacizumab*	VEGF-A and VEGFR2	Nil currently validated

Preliminary evidence on clinical, biochemical and radiological assessments | Alternate pro-angiogenic signalling circuits (eg. FGF) Bone marrow derived vascular progenitor cells & pro-angiogenic monocytes Increased pericyte coverage (Bergers & Hanahan, 2008) |
Melanoma			
Sorafenib	RAF, VEGFR, PDGFRβ, cKIT, FLT3	Nil currently validated	Alternate pro-angiogenic signalling, PDGFR mt Glucose-regulated protein 78 (Chiou et al., 2010)
Vemurafenib/ GSK 2118436	BRAF V600E/K mt	BRAF mt status	Upstream: IGF1R, PDGF upregulation, NRAS mt (Nazarian et al., 2010; Villanueva et al., 2010)) Target level: BRAF amplification, CRAF activity (Corcoran et al., 2011; Montagut et al., 2008) Downstream: MEK mt (Corcoran et al., 2011) Alternate pathway signalling: PI3K-AKT-mTOR activation
Lung Cancer			
Erlotinib/ Gefitinib	EGFR	EGFR mt status	KRAS mt EGFR T790M mt (Pao et al., 2005) EGFR insertion mt in exon 20 (Hammerman et al., 2009) EGFR trafficking (Kwak et al., 2005)

Malignancy and Drug	Target	Biomarker	Mechanisms of Resistance Under investigation
Crizotinib	ALK and MET tyrosine kinases	EML4-ALK expression on IHC, ISH and/or RT PCR	EML4-ALK with C1156Y mt EML4-ALK with L1196M mt (Choi et al., 2010)
Colorectal Cancer			
Cetuximab	EGFR	KRAS mt (codon 12)	KRAS codon 61/146 mt BRAF mt (Loupakis et al., 2009) PIK3CA mt (Sartore-Bianchi et al., 2009) PTEN loss of expression (Frattini et al., 2007)
Haematologic malignancies			
Imatinib	BCR-ABL tyrosine kinase, cKIT	BCR-ABL mRNA on PCR (peripheral blood) Cytogenetic analysis on bone marrow aspirate	Drug efflux (Mahon et al., 2003) ATP binding site mt (Branford et al., 2003) KIT mutation (in GIST) (Tamborini et al.; 2004)
CAL-101	PI3K p110δ	pAkt and markers along the PI3K δ pathway	

*Evidence for bevacizumab also applies to colorectal cancer, NSCLC, renal cell carcinoma and other malignancies
ER: estrogen receptor, PR: progesterone receptor, HER2: human epidermal growth factor receptor 2; IHC: immunohistochemistry; mt: mutation
IGF1R: insulin growth factor-1 receptor; PDGF: platelet derived growth factor
EGFR: epidermal growth factor receptor; PI3K: phosphatidylinositol-3kinase
PTEN: phosphatise and tensin homologue

Fig. 3. Selected Examples of Molecularly Targeted Therapies and Mechanisms of Drug Resistance

5.2 The breakthroughs and dilemmas of recurrent tumour biopsies

Although many mechanisms of resistance can be identified through studies of cell lines and xenograft models, it is often through correlation with patients' tumour specimens that valid conclusions can be drawn about the significance of these resistance mechanisms in the clinical setting. To this end, access to longitudinal tumour biopsies and assessment of these in 'real-time' may change the treatment paradigm for patients.

The need for longitudinal tumour biopsies is evidenced at a number of levels. Firstly, it assists in understanding and mapping the complex molecular networks, communication with the micro-environment, angiogenesis and other 'hallmarks'. As technologies in tumour analysis improve, for example with high throughput genetic sequencing and unravelling the cancer genome, findings on the pre-clinical level can be investigated and explored clinically and changes in tissue can be correlated with therapeutic response.

Secondly, there are multiple variables that can affect the accuracy of mutational analysis on tumour tissue, not least that the tumour itself can develop new mutations and aberrations that drive tumorigenesis. Studies of concordance or lack thereof, between archival primary tissue and biopsies of metastatic disease have demonstrated this in breast, colorectal and other malignancies. Analyses of HER2 over-expression in primary breast cancer and metastatic sites demonstrate that up to 12% of patients may have HER2 negative primary breast cancers with HER2 positivity at the metastatic sites, and subsequent potential therapeutic benefit from trastuzumab (Zidan et al., 2005). Conversely, up to 30% of tumours could switch from HER2 positive status on primary tissue to HER2 negative status on metastatic tissue, again significantly impacting on future treatment decisions (Locatelli et al., 2010).

In patients with advanced colorectal cancer, retrospective analyses have assessed the concordance of KRAS mutation status and other alterations along the MAPK and PI3K-AKT-mTOR pathways between primary tumours and metastatic sites. Loupakis et al. (2008) assessed PTEN status which regulates the PI3K-AKT-mTOR pathway, and demonstrated that PTEN loss occurred in 37% of tumours with associated lack of response to cetuximab and irinotecan. Interestingly the reported PTEN concordance between primary tumours and metastases was 60% compared to 95% for KRAS mutations. In those patients who were KRAS wild-type and PTEN positive on metastases, there was evidence for improved RR and PFS indicating the importance of pathway profiling to predict clinical response.

These examples underline the importance of tumour assessment not only for patients who develop metastatic disease after resection of a primary cancer, but also for patients with progressive disease on treatment. Understanding of the 'driving' pathway, receptor or network before treatment initiation, especially with new molecularly targeted agents, will become standard of care for several new treatments and guide us in the decision making algorithm even in advanced stages of disease.

This can be further evidenced by a recent study in a cohort of heavily pre-treated phase-I patients who were tested for aberrations in the MAPK and PI3K-AKT-mTOR pathways and then treated with drugs targeting these pathways (Tsimberidou et al., 2011). Impressively, those patients with molecular alterations treated with targeted therapy had a response rate of 29% (complete response or partial response) compared to 8% in the group without alterations. The proportion of patients with stable disease beyond 6 months and the median survival were also higher in this patient group.

Importantly the recent early phase-I melanoma studies with selective BRAF inhibitors have incorporated tumour biopsies at baseline, on-treatment and on-progression biopsies to analyse the changes in pathway signalling (McArthur et al., 2011; Nathanson et al., 2011). The tumour analyses included not only immunohistochemical staining, but also Sequenom MassARRAY of over 400 gene mutations, such as BRAF, RAS, PIK3CA, AKT1/2, CDK4 and others. Following this approach, patients were selected for the BRAF mutation at baseline and monitored during treatment with the measurement of phosphorylated MEK and ERK levels to confirm target inhibition. On progression, a number of potentially significant genetic alterations were identified, including NRAS and MEK1 mutations indicating continuing MAPK-pathway signalling. In addition PTEN loss and an increase in pAKT were observed, demonstrating activation of the PI3K-AKT-mTOR pathway as a possible alternate signalling pathway (Figure 2).

Clearly the risk-benefit of serial tumour biopsies needs to be well balanced and risks and disadvantages acknowledged. For example, in some cancers like NSCLC, access to tumour tissue is restricted by the site of disease with an increased potential risk of pneumothorax, bleeding and other complications secondary to a lung biopsy. Tissue biopsies also run the risk of sampling error, in part from tumour heterogeneity. As discussed with HER2 testing in gastric cancer, multiple biopsies may be required to minimise the chance of missing the alteration of interest, in this case HER2 amplification and protein over-expression. In addition sample handling, fixation, validation of assays, inter-observer variability and assessment, all contribute to the accuracy of the final result on which clinical decisions are made.

Finally, new technologies also need to be validated prior to routine introduction into clinical care. Although the ability to sequence the genome and perform genetic profiling on patients' tumours dramatically escalates the information available on an individual patient, the significance of this information is still, as yet, often unknown. The presence of a mutation does not determine its significance in tumorigenesis, such that inhibition of a given mutation will not correlate with clinical benefit, if the mutation was an incidental finding rather than an oncogenic mutation.

5.3 The role of circulating tumour cells and circulating free DNA

Detection of circulating tumour cells (CTCs), and circulating free DNA (cfDNA) in peripheral blood specimens potentially presents an easily accessible 'liquid biopsy' without the risk of tumour biopsies and further, may not only provide a predictive biomarker for a given treatment, but also contain information on molecular aberrations and changes in pathway signalling while on treatment.

There is increasing evidence that CTCs can be used as a surrogate endpoint for progression-free and overall survival and thus, allow an earlier assessment of the clinical benefit of a particular agent to streamline drug development and regulatory approval. Such 'surrogate endpoints' may accelerate drug development as long as adequate and well controlled clinical trials establish that the new drug has an effect on this surrogate, based on epidemiologic, therapeutic, pathophysiologic, or other evidence, and that this surrogate endpoint can predict clinical benefit and survival (Atkinson et al., 2001).

The enumeration of CTCs and their utility as a prognostic and predictive biomarker has been best characterised in breast, colorectal and prostate cancers with further evidence in other malignancies including melanoma and lung cancers. The most widely used and FDA approved method for CTC enumeration and molecular characterisation is the CellSearch system, which involves the immunomagnetic capture of CTCs using antibodies against the epithelial cell adhesion molecule (EpCAM), expressed on the cell surface of most epithelial malignancies. Additional cell identification includes the detection of pan-cytokeratin antibodies, DAPI nuclear staining (4,6-diamidino-2-phenylindole staining to detect nucleated cells) and CD45 negative selection to demonstrate the detected cell is not a leucocyte.

The presence of CTCs at baseline in metastatic breast cancer has not only been demonstrated to have prognostic significance but has also been shown to be the strongest predictor of overall survival when compared to age, hormone receptor status, HER2 status and metastatic site. It also maintains its prognostic value independent of line of treatment, site of recurrence and disease phenotype (Cristofanilli et al., 2005). Preliminary studies in breast cancer suggest that CTC enumeration may even be superior to radiological evaluation in predicting response to treatment and outcome. It may provide a more reproducible indication of disease status compared to current imaging methods, particularly in view of inter-reader variability in confirming radiological response which can vary by up to 15% compared to 1% variability for CTC counts (Budd et al., 2006).

In castrate resistant prostate cancer, the presence of CTCs at baseline and lack of a decline during treatment is also indicative of poor response and survival. In multivariate analyses, CTC counts and PSA doubling time have been demonstrated as the only independent predictors for clinical outcome as compared to PSA level, Gleason Score, bone metastases and age (De Bono et al., 2008). Additionally, there is now evidence that CTCs may be a potential surrogate biomaker in metastatic prostate cancer trials. The randomised, double-blind phase III trial in metastatic prostate cancer, in which abiraterone was compared to placebo, was the first of its kind to demonstrate the utility of CTCs in this setting. CTCs were measured at baseline and repeated at 4, 8 and 12 weeks post treatment. Pre-treatment CTCs were strongly correlated with OS, as was a fall in CTC count on treatment (Reid et al., 2010; Scher et al., 2011). Particularly in the setting of castrate resistant prostate cancer where there may be inter-observer variation regarding radiological progression, CTCs may provide an accurate and reproducible alternative.

In patients with metastatic colorectal cancer, higher baseline CTC counts correlate with shorter PFS and OS. Again, conversion of an unfavourable baseline CTC count to a favourable count at 3-5 weeks after starting treatment is associated with longer PFS and OS compared with patients with unfavourable counts at both time points. Baseline and follow-up CTC levels also remain strong predictors of PFS and OS after adjustment for clinically significant factors (Cohen et al., 2008).

Recent evaluation of CTCs in patients with NSCLC has also suggested prognostic significance (Krebs et al., 2011). CTCs in patients with NSCLC were found more commonly with stage IV (32%) compared to stage IIIB disease (7%) and in those patients with five or more CTCs detected, both PFS and OS were inferior. Particularly with the complexities in obtaining longitudinal tissue biopsies, further investigation of a prognostic 'liquid biopsy' and incorporation into early phase trials is of importance.

In patients with advanced melanoma, recent studies have demonstrated good correlation between CTC status and tumor-node-metastasis stage, underlining the prognostic role of CTCs (Mocellin et al., 2006). The predictive value of CTCs was so far limited by the fact that treatment options consisted of bio-chemotherapies with no effects on clinical outcomes. However, the presence of circulating melanoma cells after adjuvant treatment for stage III melanoma has been shown to correlate with inferior relapse-free and overall survival and may be a useful indicator of systemic subclinical disease (Koyanagi et al., 2005). Isolation and molecular characterisation of these cells, combined with analysis of cfDNA, presents an opportunity to obtain further information about the pathways driving tumorigenesis, invasion and metastasis. In addition to evaluating the role of CTCs in melanoma, one study found good correlation between CTCs and cfDNA suggesting both markers may be a useful determinant of disease status and treatment effect. Patients with measurable CTC or cfDNA showed poorer disease outcome compared with patients without these markers, and patients with both markers showed the most inferior disease outcome, despite the fact that the treatment regimens were heterogenous and consisted of bio-chemotherapies of limited clinical benefit (Koyanagi et al., 2006).

5.4 Optimising trial design

Given the diversity of novel compounds discovered over the last decade, clinical trial design for the evaluation of these targeted agents has evolved with the agents being tested. Many of these agents do not cause typical chemotherapy-induced side effects such as myelosupression around which early phase trial design has been based. Therefore design of clinical trials of novel agents has had to develop in order to evaluate these agents appropriately and efficiently.

In a standard dose escalation phase I trial, cohorts of three to six patients are treated at pre-defined dose levels, dose-limiting toxicity (DLT) is observed and the maximum tolerated dose (MTD) is defined as the dose level where >33% of patients treated have experienced a DLT. Dose levels are commonly defined using modification of the original Fibonacci design (increasing dose by fixed increments of 100%, 67%, 50%, 40% followed by 33% for all subsequent levels) but slow attainment of the MTD and exposure of significant numbers of patients to low doses have been criticisms of this approach (Rogatko et al, 2007). An accelerated trial design (Simon et al, 1997) is now a widely accepted alternative to the Fibonacci dose-definition model and many trials now allow individual patients to be dose-escalated within a study if safe to do so, aiming to minimise those being exposed to ineffective doses. Therefore there are many combinations of model-based and rule-based designs that allow flexibility of the recruitment structure in a trial and can be appropriately adapted to the agent under consideration (Ivy et al., 2010; Parulekar et al., 2004; Rogatko et al, 2005; Korn et al, 2001; Cannistra et al., 2008; Sleijfer et al., 2008; Bria et al., 2009).

The appropriateness of the primary endpoint of maximum tolerated dose (MTD) has been challenged for some of these agents and consideration has been given instead to the concept of optimal biological dose (OBD) (O'Reilly et al., 2010; Le Tourneau et al., 2009). Targeted biological agents are more commonly cystostatic rather than cytotoxic, therefore other endpoints should be considered when evaluating treatment efficacy (Rixe et al., 2007; Gelmon et al., 1999) including novel radiographic assessment and immunotherapy assessment (Wolchok et al., 2009).

There has also been an increasing realization that patients need to be appropriately selected for certain agents based on tumour biology and molecular characteristics. The question is whether patient selection should take place at the outset of drug development, as a targeted approach which is then diversified; or whether a broader recruitment strategy should prevail initially, followed by testing within a targeted population. There is therefore a critical need to integrate and validate novel biomarkers into drug development from the earliest stages of evaluation, incorporating tumour and non-tumour tissue samples to apply these biomarkers appropriately and guide patient selection.

Overall, in the era of development of molecularly targeted agents, appropriately designed hypothesis-testing trials should be conducted. Patients should be selected rationally according to tumour biology and molecular characteristics and above all, an element of flexibility should be allowed within the trial design to enable response to unexpected findings, whether that be toxicity or efficacy.

6. Conclusion

The increased understanding of tumour biology and genetics along with improvements in laboratory methodologies and IT-systems will continue to make a tremendous impact on oncology drug development. Critical to future oncology drug development is the incorporation of biomarkers from the earliest stages and supported by applied bioinformatics. In addition, the use of new preclinical models and novel clinical trial designs incorporating intermediate surrogate biomarker endpoints will be essential not only for the better understanding of mechanisms of action of new targeted drugs, but also in supporting confident *'go or no-go decisions'*. The *'personalised medicine'* approach involving molecular characterisation of the tumour and its context within the micro-environment and immune system, will help to define the right treatment, for the right patient at the right time. Increasing our understanding on how to combine established and novel therapeutics in an efficient timeframe is critical to improved outcomes for the treatment of solid malignancies.

7. Acknowledgments

Diagrams were designed with the assistance of Sabina Pasha, Sarah Cannon Research UK.

8. References

Albarello, L.; Pecciarini, L. & Doglioni, C. (2011) HER2 testing in gastric cancer. *Advances in Anatomic Pathology;* 18(1): 53-59.

Bang, Y-J.; Van Cutsem, E. ; Feyereislova, A. ; et al. (2010) Trastuzumab in combination with chemotherapy versus chemotherapy alone for treatment of HER2-positive advanced gastric or gastro-oesophageal junction cancer (ToGA): a phase 3, open-label, randomised controlled trial. *Lancet;* 376 (9742): 687-697.

Bartlett, M.S.; Going, J.J.; Mallon, E.A.; et al. (2001) Evaluating HER2 amplification and overexpression in breast cancer. *The Journal of Path;* 195 (4): 422-428.

Batchelor, T.T.; Sorensen, A.G.; di Tomasi, E.; et al. (2007) AZD2171, a pan-VEGF receptor tyrosine kinase inhibitor, normalizes tumor vasculature and alleviates edema in glioblastoma patients. *Cancer Cell;* 11: 83-95.

Bergers, G. & Hanahan, D. (2008) Modes of resistance to anti-angiogenic therapy. *Nature Reviews;* 8: 592-603.

Atkinson, A.J.; Colburn, W.A.; DeGruttola, V.G.; et al. (2001) Biomarkers and surrogate endpoints: preferred definitions and conception framework. *Clin Pharmacol Ther;* 69: 89-95.

Bocci, G.; Man, S.; Green, S.K.; et al. (2004) Increased plasma vascular endothelial growth factor (VEGF) as a surrogate marker for optimal therapeutic dosing of VEGF receptor-2 monoclonal antibodies. *Cancer Res;* 64: 6616-6625.

Branford, S. ; Rudzki, Z. ; Walsh, S. ; et al. (2003) Detection of BCR-ABL mutations in patients with CML treated with imatinib is virtually always accompanied by clinical resistance, and mutations in the ATP phosphate-binding loop (P-loop) are associated with poor prognosis. *Blood* ; 102 (1) : 276-283.

Bria, E.; Di Maio, M.; Carlini, P.; et al. (2009) Targeting targeted agents: Open issues for clinical trial design. *J Exp Clin Cancer Res;* 28: 66.

Budd, G.T. ; Cristofanilli, M. ; Ellis, M.J. ; et al. (2006) Circulating tumour cells versus imaging – predicting overall survival in metastatic breast cancer. *Clin Cancer Res;* 12: 6403-6409.

Cannistra, S.A. (2008) Challenges and pitfalls of combining targeted agents in phase i studies. *J Clin Oncol;* 26(22): 3665-3667.

Cappuzzo, F. ; Ciuleanu, T.; Stelmakh, L.; et al. (2010) Erlotinib as maintenance treatment in advanced non-small-cell lung cancer: a multicentre, randomised, placebo-controlled phase 3 study. *The Lancet Oncology;* 11(6): 521-529.

Carlson, B. (2008) HER2 Tests: How Do We Choose? *Biotechnology Healthcare*; Sept/Oct edition: 23-27.

Casanovas, O.; Hicklin, D.J.; Bergers, G. & Hanahan, D. (2005) Drug resistance by evasion of antiangiogenic targeting of VEGF signaling in late-stage pancreatic islet tumours. *Cancer Cell*; 8: 299-309.

Chapman, P.B.; Hauschild, A.; Robert, C.; et al. (2011) Improved survival with vemurafenib in melanoma with BRAF V600E mutation. *New Engl J Med*; June (10.1056/NEJMoa1103782).

Chiou, J-F.; Tai, C-J.; Huang, M-T. ; et al. (2010) Glucose-regulated proteint 78 is a novel contributor to acquisition of resistance to sorafenib in hepatocellular carcinoma. *Ann Surg Oncol*; 17(2): 603-612.

Choi, Y.L.; Soda, M.; Yamashita, Y.; et al. (2010) EML4-ALK mutations in lung cancer that confer resistance to ALK inhibitors. New Engl J Med; 363: 1734-1739.

Cohen, S.J.; Punt, C.J.; Iannotti, N.; et al (2008) Relationship of circulating tumor cells to tumor response, progression-free survival, and overall survival in patients with metastatic colorectal cancer. *J Clin Oncol*; 26(19): 3213-21.

Corcoran, R.B.; Dias-Santagata, D.; Bergethon, K.; et al. (2010) BRAF gene amplification can promote acquired resistance to MEK inhibitors in cancer cells harbouring the BRAF V600E mutation. *Sci Signal* 3: ra84.

Corcoran, R.B.; Settleman, J. & Engelman, J.A. (2011) Potential Therapetuic Strategies to overcome Acquired Resistance to BRAF or MEK inhibitors in BRAF mutant cancers. *Oncotarget* 2(4): 336-346.

Cristofanilli, M. ; Hayes, D.F. ; Budd, G.T. ; et al. (2005) Circulating Tumour cells : a novel prognostic factor for newly diagnosed metastic breast cancer. *J Clin Oncol*; 23(7): 1420-1430.

Cunningham, D.; Humblet, Y.; Siena, S.; et al. (2004) Cetuximab monotherapy and cetuximab plus irinotecan in irinotecan-refractory metastatic colorectal cancer. *New Engl J Med*; 351(4): 337-45.

Davies, H. ; Bignell, G.R. ; Cox, C. ; et al. (2002) Mutations of the BRAF gene in human cancer. *Nature* 417: 949-954.

De Bono, J.S.; Scher, H.I.; Montgomery, R.B.; et al. (2008) Circulating tumor cells predict survival benefit from treatment in metastatic castration-resistant prostate cancer. *Clin Cancer Res*; 14(9):6302-6309.

De Bono, J.S. & Ashworth, A. (2010) Translating cancer research into targeted therapeutics. *Nature*; 467: 543-549.

De Roock, W.; Jonker, D.J.; Di Nicolantonio, F.; et al. (2010) Association of KRAS p.G13D Mutation with outcome in patients with chemotherapy-refractory metastatic colorectal cancer treated with cetuximab. *JAMA*; 304(16): 1812-1820.

Eisen, T.; Ahmad, T.; Flaherty, K.T.; et al. (2006) Sorafenib in advanced melanoma : a Phase II randomised discontinuation trial analysis. *Br J of Cancer* 95: 581-586.

Emery, C.M.; Vijayendram, K.G.; Zipser, M.C.; et al. (2009) MEK1 mutations confer resistance to MEK and BRAF inhibition. *Proc Natl Acad Sci USA* 106(48): 20411-20416.

Escudier, B.; Szczylik, C.; Eisen, T.; et al. (2005) Randomized phase III trial of the multi-kinase inhibitor BAY 43-9006 in patients with advanced renal cell carcinoma. *Eur J Cancer Suppls*; 3: 226.

Flaherty, K.T.; Puzanov, I.; Kim, K.B.; et al. (2010) Inhibition of Mutated, Activated BRAF in Metastatic Melanoma. *New Engl J Med* 363(9): 809-819.

Flinn, I.W.; Byrd, J.C.; Furman, R.R.; et al. (2009) Preliminary evidence of clinical activity in a phase I study of CAL-101, a selective inhibitor of the p110δ isoform of phosphatidylinositol 3-kinase (PI3K), in patients with select haematologic malignancies. *J Clin Oncol*; 27: 15s (suppl; abstr 3543)

Frattini, M.; Saletti, P.; Romagnani, E.; et al. (2007) PTEN loss of expression predicts cetuximab efficacy in metastatic colorectal cancer patients. *Br J Cancer*; 97: 1139-1145.

Fukuoka, M.; Wu, Y-L.; Thongprasert, S. ; et al. (2011) Biomarker Analyses and Final Overall Survival Results from a phase III, randomised, open-label, first-line study of gefitinib versus carboplatin/paclitaxel in clinically selected patients with advanced non-small cell lung cancer in Asia (IPASS). *J Clin Oncol*, published online June 13: doi 10.1200/JCO.2010.33.4235.

Gelmon, K.A.; Eisenhauer, E.A.; Harris, A.L.; et al. (1999) Anticancer agents targeting signaling molecules and cancer cell environment: Challenges for drug development? *J Natl Cancer Inst*; 91(15): 1281-1287.

Gottesman, M.M. (2002) Mechanisms of Cancer Drug Resistance. Annu Rev Med; 53: 615-27.

Gysin, S.; Salt, M.; Young, A. & McCormick, F. (2011) Therapeutic Strategies for Targeting Ras proteins. *Genes & Cancer*; 2(3): 359-372.

Hammerman, P.S.; Jänne, P.A. & Johnson, B.E. (2009) Resistance to Epidermal Growth Factor Receptor Tyrosine Kinase Inhibitors in Non-Small Cell Lung Cancer. *Clin Can Res*; 15: 7502-7509.

Hanahan, D. & Folkman, J. (1996) Patterns and emerging mechanisms of the angiogenic switch during tumorigenesis. *Cell*: 86: 353-364.

Hanahan, D. & Weinberg, R.A. (2011) Hallmarks of Cancer: The Next Generation. Cell; 144: 646-669.

Hanahan, D. & Weinberg, R.A. (2000) The hallmarks of cancer. *Cell* 100; 57-70.

Hauschild, A., Agarwala, S.S.; Trefzer, U.; et al. (2009) Results of a phase III, randomized placebo-controlled study of sorafenib in combination with carboplatin and paclitaxel as second-line treatment in patients with unresectable stage III or IV melanoma. *J Clin Oncol* 27(17): 2823-2830.

Herman, S.E.M.; Gordon, A.L.; Wagner, A.J.; et al. (2010) Phosphatidylinositol 3-kinase- δ inhibitor CAL-101 shows promising preclinical activity in chronic lymphocytic leukaemia by antagonizing intrinsic and extrinsic cellular survival signals. *Blood*; 116(12): 2078-2088.

Hofmann, M.; Stoss, O.; Gaiser, T.; et al. (2008a) Central HER2 IHC and FISH analysis in a trastuzumab (Herceptin) phase II monotherapy study: assessment of test sensitivity and impact of chromosome 17 polysomy. *J Clin Pathol*; 61(1): 89-94.

Hofmann, M.; Stoss, O.; Shi, D.; et al. (2008b) Assessment of a HER2 scoring system for gastric cancer: results from a validation study. *Histopathology*; 52: 797–805

Houben, R.; Becker, J.C.; Kappel, A.; et al. (2004) Constitutive activation of the Ras-Raf signalling pathway in metastatic melanoma is associated with poor prognosis. *J of Carcinogenesis* 3 (1): 6.

Hurwitz, H; Fehrenbacher, L; Novotny, W; et al. (2004) Bevacizumab plus irinotecan, fluorouracil and leucovorin for metastatic colorectal cancer. *N Engl J Med*; 350(23): 2335-42.

Ivy, S.P.; Garrett-Mayer, E. & Rubinstein, L. (2010) Approaches to phase 1 clinical trial design focused on safety, efficiency, and selected patient populations: a report from the clinical trial design task force of the national cancer institute investigational drug steering committee. *Clin Cancer Res*.;16(6):1726-36.

Jakob, J.A.; Bassett, R.L.; Ng, C.S.; et al. (2011) Clinical characteristics and outcomes associated with BRAF and NRAS mutations in metastatic melanoma. *J Clin Oncol* 29 (suppl; abstr 8500)

Jiang, C.C. ; Lai, F. ; Thorne, R.F. ; et al. (2011) MEK-independent survival of B-RAF V600E melanoma cells selected for resistance to apoptosis induced by the RAF inhibitor PLX4720. *Clin Cancer Res* 17: 721-730.

Jubb, A.M.; Harris, A.L. (2010) Biomarkers to predict the clinical efficacy of bevacizumab in cancer. *Lancet Oncol*; 11: 1172-83.

Karapetis, C.S. ; Khambata-Ford, S. ; Jonker, D.J.; et al. (2008) K-ras mutations and benefit from cetuximab in advanced colorectal cancer. *New Engl J Med*; 359(17): 1757-65.

Karasarides, M.; Chiloeches, A.; Hayward, R.; et al. (2004) B-RAF is a therapeutic target in melanoma. *Oncogene* 23; 6292-6298.

Kefford, R.; Arkenau, H.; Brown, M.P.; et al. (2010) Phase I/II study of GSK2118436, a selective inhibitor of oncogenic mutant BRAF kinase, in patients with metastatic melanoma and other solid tumours. *J Clin Oncol* 28: 15s (suppl; abstr 8503).

Kobayashi, S. ; Ji, H. ; Yuza, Y. ; et al. (2005) An Alternative inhibitor overcomes resistance caused by a mutation of the epidermal growth factor receptor. *Cancer Res*; 65: 7096-7101.

Korn, E.L.; Arbuck, S.G.; Pluda, J.M.; et al. (2001) Clinical trial designs for cytostatic agents: Are new approaches needed? *J Clin Oncol*; 19(1): 265-272.

Koyanagi, K.; O'Day, S.J.; Gonzalez, R.; et al (2005) Serial Monitoring of circulating melanoma cells during neoadjuvant biochemotherapy for stage III melanoma: outcome prediction in a multicenter trial. *J Clin Oncol*; 23(31): 8057-8064.

Koyanagi, K. ; Mori, T. ; O'Day, S.; et al. (2006) Association of Circulating Tumour Cells with Serum Tumor-Related Methylated DNA in peripheral blood of melanoma patients. *Cancer Res*; 66: 6111-6117.

Krebs, M.G.; Sloane, R.; Priest, L.; et al. (2011) Evaluation and Prognostic Significance of Circulating Tumor cells in patients with non-small-cell lung cancer. *J Clin Oncol*; 29(12): 1556-1563.

Kwak, E.L.; Bang, Y-J.; Camidge, R.; et al. (2010) Anaplastic Lymphona Kinase inhibition in non-small-cell lung cancer. *N Engl J Med*, 363 (18): 1693-1703.

Kwak, E.L.; Sordella, R.; Bell, D.W.; et al. (2005) Irreversible inhibitors of the EGF receptor may circumvent acquired resistance to gefitinib. *Proc Nat Acad Sci*; 102 (21): 7665-7670

Lannutti, B.J.; Meadows, S.A.; Herman, S.E.M.; et al. (2011) CAL-101, a p110 δ selective phosphatidylinositol-3-kinase inhibitor for the treatment of B-cell malignancies inhibits PI3K signalling and cellular viability. *Blood*; 117(2): 591-594.

Le Tourneau, C.; Lee, J.J.; Siu, L.L. (2009) Dose escalation methods in phase I cancer clinical trials. *J Natl Cancer Inst*; 101(10): 708-720.

Lievre, A.; Bachet, J-B.; Le Corre, D. ; et al. (2006) KRAS mutation status is predictive of response to cetuximab therapy in colorectal cancer. *Cancer Res*; 66(8): 3992-3995.

Little, A.S.; Balmanno, K.; Sale, M.J.; et al. (2011) Amplification of the Driving Oncogene, KRAS or BRAF, Underpins Acquired Resistance to MEK1/2 Inhibitors in Colorectal Cancer Cells. *Sci Signal* 4: ra17.

Llovet, J.M.; Ricci, S.; Mazzaferro, V.; et al. Sorafenib in advanced hepatocellular carcinoma. *New Engl J Med*; 359: 378-380.

Locatelli, M.A.; Curigliano, G.; Fumagalli, L.; et al. (2010) Should liver metastases of breast cancer be biopsied to improve treatment choice? *J Clin Onc*; 28: 18s (suppl; abstr CRA1008)

Long, G.V.; Menzies, A.M.; Nagrial, A.M.; et al. (2011) Prognostic and clinicopathologic associations of oncogenic BRAF in metastatic melanoma. *J Clin Oncol* 29(10): 1239-1246.

Loupakis, F.; Pollina, L.; Stasi, I.; et al. (2008) Evaluation of PTEN expression in colorectal cancer (CRC) metastases (mets) and in primary tumors as predictors of activity of cetuximab plus irinotecan treatment. *J Clin Oncol*; 26: 15S (abstr 4003).

Loupakis, F.; Ruzzo, A.; Cremolini, C.; et al. (2009) KRAS codon 61,146 and BRAF mutations predict resistance to cetuximab plus irinotecan in KRAS codon 12 and 13 wild-type metastatic colorectal cancer. *Br J Cancer*; 101: 715-721.

Lu, Y.H.; Zi, X.; Zhao, Y.; et al. (2001) Insulin-like growth-factor-1 receptor signalling and resistance to trastuzumab (Herceptin). *J Natl Cancer Inst*; 93: 1852-1857.

Mahon, F.X.; Belloc, F.; Lagarde, V.; et al. (2003) MDR1 gene overexpression confers resistance to imatinib mesylate in leukemia cell line models. *Blood*; 101: 2368–2373.

McArthur, G.; Ribas, A.; Chapman, P.B.; et al. (2011) Molecular analyses from a Phase 1 trial of vemurafenib to study mechanism of action and resistance in repeated biopsies from BRAF mutation positive metastatic melanoma patients. *J Clin Oncol* 29 (suppl, abstr 8502).

Mocellin, S.; Hoon, D.; Ambrosi, A.; et al. (2006) The Prognostic Value of Circulating Tumor Cells in Patients with Melanoma: A Systematic Review and Meta-analysis. *Clin Cancer Res*; 12: 4605-4613

Montagut, C.; Sharma, S.V.; Shioda, T.; et al. (2008) Elevated CRAF as a potential mechanism of acquired resistance to BRAF inhibition in melanoma. *Cancer Res* 68: 4853-4861.

Nagy, P.; Friedlander, E.; Tanner, M.; et al. (2005) Decreased accessibility and lack of activation of ErbB2 in JIMT-1, a herceptin-resistant, MUC4-expressing breast cancer cell line. *Cancer Res*; 65: 473-482.

Nathanson, K.L.; Martin, A.; Letrero, R.; et al. (2011) Tumor genetic analyses of patients with metastatic melanoma treated with the BRAF inhibitor GSK2118436 (GSK436). *J Clin Oncol* 29: (suppl; abstr 8501)

Nazarian, R.; Shi, H.; Wang, Q.; et al. (2010) Melanomas acquire resistance to B-RAF (V600E) inhibition by RTK or N-RAS upregulation. *Nature* 468: 973-977.

O'Reilly, T.; McSheehy, P.M.; Kawai, R.; et al. (2010) Comparative pharmacokinetics of RAD001 in normal and tumor-bearing rodents. *Cancer Chemother Pharmacol*; 65(4): 625-39.

Paik, S.; Bryant, J.; Tan-Chiu, E.; et al. (2002) Real-world performance of HER2 testing-National Surgical Adjuvant Breast and Bowel Project experience. *J Natl Cancer Inst*; 94: 852-854.

Pao, W.; Miller, V.A.; Politi, K.A.; Riely, G.J.; Somwar, R.; et al. (2005) Acquired Resistance of Lung Adenocarcinomas to Gefitinib or Erlotinib Is Associated with a Second Mutation in the EGFR Kinase Domain. *PLoS Med* 2(3): e73. doi:10.1371/journal.pmed.0020073

Paraiso, K.H.T. ; Xiang, Y. ; Rebecca, V.W. ; et al. (2011) PTEN loss confers BRAF inhibitor resistance to melanoma cells through the suppression of BIM expression. *Cancer Res* 71(7): 2750-2760.

Parulekar, W.R. & Eisenhauer, E.A. (2004) Phase i trial design for solid tumor studies of targeted, non-cytotoxic agents: Theory and practice. *J Natl Cancer Inst;* 96(13): 990-997.

Platz, A.; Egyhazi, S.; Ringborg, U.; et al. (2008) Human cutaneous melanoma; a review of NRAS and BRAF mutation frequencies in relation to histogenic subclass and body site. *Mol Oncol* 1: 395-405.

Relf, M. ; LeJeune, S. ; Scott, P.A. ; et al. (1997) Expression of the angiogenic factors vascular endothelial cell growth factor, acidic and basic fibroblast growth factor, tumor growth factor beta-1, platelet-derived endothelial cell growth factor, placenta growth factor and pleiotrophin in human primary bresat cancer and its relation to angiogenesis. *Cancer Res;* 57: 963-969.

Reid, A.H.M.; Attard, G.; Danila, D.C.; et al (2010) Significant and Sustained antitumor activity in post-docetaxel, castration-resistant prostate cancer with the CYP17 inhibitor abiraterone acetate. *J Clin Onc;* 28(9): 1489-1495.

Ribas, A.; Kim, K.B.; Schuchter, L.M.; et al. (2011) BRIM-2: an open-label, multicenter phase II study of vemurafenib in previously treated patients with BRAFV600E mutation-positive melanoma. *J Clin Oncol* 29: Suppl:8509-8509.

Ring, A. & Dowsett, M. (2004) Mechanisms of tamoxifen resistance. *Endocr Relat Cancer;* 11: 643-658,

Rixe, O. & Fojo, T. (2007) Is cell death a critical end point for anticancer therapies or is cytostasis sufficient? *Clin Cancer Res:* 13(24): 7280-7287.

Robert, J. (1999) Multidrug resistance in oncology: diagnostic and therapeutic approaches. *Eur J of Clin Inv;* 29: 536-545.

Roche, P.C.; Suman, V.J.; Jenkins, R.B.; et al. (2002) Concordance between local and central laboratory HER2 testing in the breast intergroup trial N9831. *J Natl Cancer Inst ;* 94:855-857.

Rogatko, A.; Babb, J.S.; Tighiouart, M.; et al. (2005) New paradigm in dose-finding trials: Patient-specific dosing and beyond phase I. *Clin Cancer Res;* 11(15): 5342-5346.

Rogatko, A.; Schoeneck, D.; Jonas, W.; et al. (2007) Translation of innovative designs into phase i trials. *J Clin Oncol;* 25(31): 4982-4986.

Romond, E.H. ; Perez, E.A. ; Bryant, J. ; et al. (2005) Trastuzumab plus adjuvant chemotherapy for operable HER2-positive breast cancer. *N Engl J Med;*353:1673-1684

Rosell, R. ; Gervais, R. ; Vergnenegre, A. ; et al. (2011) Erlotinib versus chemotherapy in advanced non-small cell lung cancer (NSCLC) patients with epidermal growth factor receptor mutations: interim results of the European Erlotinib Versus Chemotherapy (EURTAC) phase III randomized trial. *J Clin Oncol;* 29: (suppl; abstr 7503).

Sartore-Bianchi, A.; Martini, M.; Molinari, F.; et al. (2009) PIK3CA mutations in colorectal cancer are associated with clinical resistance to EGFR-targeted monoclonal antibodies. *Cancer Res;* 69: 1851-1857.

Scher, H.I.; Heller, G.; Molina, A.; et al. (2011) Evaluation of circulating tumour cell (CTC) enumeration as an efficacy response biomarker of overall survival (OS) in metastatic castration-resistance prostate cancer (mCRPC): Planned final analysis (FA) of COU-AA-301, a randomized double-blind, placebo-controlled phase III study of abiraterone acetate (AA) plus low-dose prednisone (P) post docetaxel. *J Clin Oncol*; 29: suppl (abstr LBA4517)

Shao, Y.; Aplin, A.E. (2010) Akt3-mediated resistance to apoptosis in BRAF-targeted melanoma cells. *Cancer Res* 70(16): 6670-6681.

Shepherd, F.A. ; Pereira, J.R. ; Ciuleanu, T. ; et al. (2005) Erlotinib in Previouly Treated Non-Small-Cell Lung Cancer. *N Engl J Med*; 353: 123-132.

Simon, R.; Freedman, L.S.; (1997) Bayesian design and analysis of two x two factorial clinical trials. *Biometrics*; 53(2): 456-464.

Slamon, D.J.; Clark, G.M.; Wong, S.G.; et al. (1987) Human breast cancer : correlation of relapse and survival with amplification of the HER-2/neu oncogene. *Science (Wash DC)*; 235: 177-182.

Slamon, D.J. ; Godolphin, W. ; Jones, L.A. ; et al. (1989) Studies of the HER-2/neu proto-oncogene in human breast and ovarian cancer. *Science*; 244: 707-712.

Slamon, D.J.; Leyland-Jones, B.; Shak, S.; et al. (2001)Use of chemotherapy plus a monoclonal antibody against HER2 for metastatic breast cancer that overexpresses HER2. *N Engl J Med*; 344: 783-792

Sleijfer, S, & Wiemer, E. (2008) Dose selection in phase I studies: Why we should always go for the top. *J Clin Oncol*; 26(10): 1576-1578.

Szakacs, G.; Paterson, J.K.; Ludwig, J.A.; et al. (2006) Targeting multidrug resistance in cancer. *Nature Reviews*; 5: 219-234.

Tamborini, E.; Bonadiman, L.; Greco, A.; et al. (2004) A new mutation in the KIT ATP pocket causes acquired resistance to imatinib in a gastrointestinal stromal tumor patient. *Gastroenterology*; 127(1): 294-299.

Thatcher, N.; Chang, A.; Parikh, P.; et al. (2005) Gefitinib plus best supportive care in patients with refractory advanced non-small-cell lung cancer: results from a randomised, placebo-controlled, multicentre study (Iressa Survival Evaluation in Lung Cancer). *Lancet*; 366: 1527-1537.

Tsimberidou, A.M.; Iskander, N.G.; Hong, D.S.; et al. (2011) Personalized medicine in a phase 1 clinical trials program: The M.D. Anderson Cancer Center Initiative. *J Clin Oncol*; 29: (suppl; abstr CRA2500)

Villanueva, J. ; Vultur, A. ; Lee, J.T. ; et al. (2010) Acquired resistance to BRAF inhibitors mediated by a RAF kinase switch in melanoma can be overcome by targeting MEK and IGF-1R/PI3K. *Cancer Cell* 18: 683-695.

Wagle, N.; Emery, C.; Berger, M.F.; et al. (2011) Dissecting Therapeutic Resistance to RAF inhibition in melanoma by Tumor Genomic Profiling. *J Clin Oncol* published online on March 7, 2011 (DOI:10.1200/JCO.2010.33.2312).

Wiley, H.S. (2003) Trafficking of the ErbB receptors and its influence on signalling. *Exp Cell Res*; 284: 78-88.

Wilhelm, C.; Carter, C.; Lynch, M.; et al. (2006) Discovery and development of sorafenib: A multikinase inhibitor for treating cancer. *Nat Rev Drug Discov*; 5: 835-44.

Wolchok, J.D.; Hoos, A.; O'Day, S.; et al. (2009) Guidelines for the evaluation of immune therapy activity in solid tumors: immune-related response criteria. *Clin. Cancer Res*; 15(23): 7412–7420.

Wolff, A.C.; Hammond, E.H.; Schwartz, J.N.; et al. (2007) American Society of Clinical Oncology/College of American Pathologists Guideline Recommendations for Human Epidermal Growth Factor Receptor 2 Testing in Breast Cancer. *J Clin Oncol*; 25(1): 118-145.

Yano, T. ; Doi, T. ; Ohtsu, A. ; et al. (2006) Comparison of HER2 gene amplification assessed by fluorescence in situ hybridization and HER2 protein expression assessed by immunohistochemistry in gastric cancer. *Oncol Rep*; 15: 65-71.

Zidan, J.; Dashkovsky, I.; Stayerman, C.; et al. (2005) Comparison of HER2 overexpression in primary breast cancer and metastatic sites and its effect on biological targeting therapy of metastatic disease. *Br J Cancer*; 93: 552-556.

Part 2

Models

5

Genetic Pharmacotherapy

Celia Gellman[1,2], Susana Mingote[1,2], Yvonne Wang[1,2],
Inna Gaisler-Salomon[1,3] and Stephen Rayport[1,2]
[1]Department of Psychiatry, Columbia University
[2]Department of Molecular Therapeutics, New York State Psychiatric Institute
[3]Department of Psychology, University of Haifa
USA

1. Introduction

In current drug development, *proof-of-concept*—determining whether a ligand engaging its target is likely to be therapeutic—requires specific ligands. This presents a catch-22, as the motivation to develop ligands requires proof-of-concept studies that cannot be conducted without ligands. A strategy we term *genetic pharmacotherapy*—a refinement of genetic blockade focused on druggable targets—obviates the catch-22 by enabling proof-of-concept studies *prior* to the development of specific ligands via genetic means in mouse models. In this strategy, which could help avert investment in molecular entities that will ultimately prove therapeutically inefficacious, a gene is conditionally down-regulated via a molecular *switch* in adult mice. Both the precise temporal control of the intervention and the consequent change in target protein function parallel the administration of drugs, with the additional advantage of perfect specificity. Moreover genetic pharmacotherapy overcomes the impediment of the blood-brain barrier, which makes developing ligands for psychiatric disorders particularly challenging. Here, we describe the transgenic technologies that form the basis for the strategy, discuss the advantages and limitations in juxtaposition with other gene expression modification approaches, contrast examples of prior implementation, address the feasibility for systematic use, and illustrate past and future opportunities. Although the molecular tools are widely available, genetic pharmacotherapy has only been implemented outside the central nervous system (CNS), despite its particular utility for CNS disorders. The systematic application of this strategy should foster the development of new, innovative molecular therapies.

2. The conceptual basis and requisite components of genetic pharmacotherapy

We define genetic pharmacotherapy as the use of a genetic intervention to achieve a pharmacological effect. Genetic pharmacotherapy has two requirements. First, genetic blockade must be universal — reaching all cells in the body, including the brain — to simulate organism-wide drug distribution. Second, induction of gene-modulation must be temporally controllable, as opposed to originating during embryogenesis, so that target modulation occurs as it would with drug administration. While traditional knockout strategies have been used extensively to study the roles of proteins in a broad range of disorders, constitutive mutations are often lethal in early life precluding study of target gene function in adulthood (Lewandoski, 2001). Moreover, many non-lethal knockouts of genes of interest elicit paradoxical phenotypes — phenotypes that are opposite to the effects of pharmacologic blockade of the same target in adulthood — as a result of developmental compensations (Gingrich & Hen, 2000). The genetic strategy that satisfies these two requirements is a refinement of Cre-lox recombination, in which two individually silent mutations are introduced. One mutation drives a ligand-inducible effector enzyme that enables target-modulation, and the other mutation makes the target gene of interest susceptible to inactivation by the effector enzyme. This involves breeding a mouse carrying the inducible effector — CreERT — with an animal carrying the effector-sensitized *floxed* gene-of-interest. In the resulting progeny, inducing the CreERT produces irreversible target modulation paralleling the institution of pharmacotherapy.

2.1 Origins of the inducible-Cre strategy

In Cre-lox recombination, Cre recombinase — from P1 bacteriophage — recognizes two closely spaced 34-base pair loxP sequences, excises the intervening sequence, and recombines the flanking strands. When placed strategically by homologous recombination, the excision inactivates the so-called floxed gene (Nagy, 2000; Sternberg & Hamilton, 1981) (**Figure 1a**). To inactivate the target gene, a mouse that carries the Cre transgene is bred with a mouse carrying loxP sites flanking a portion of the gene of interest (the floxed gene); in the resulting F_1 progeny the floxed gene is inactivated in all cells where Cre is expressed (**Figure 1b**).

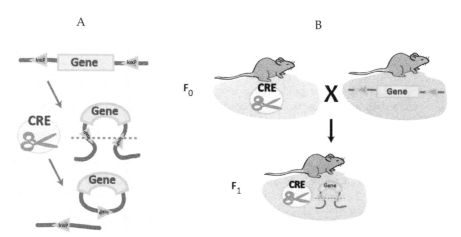

Fig. 1. Removal of targeted DNA sequences by Cre-lox recombination. A. Cre recombinase excises the portion of DNA between the loxP recognition sites (the floxed gene), recombining the flanking strands. B. To accomplish this in mice, a mouse carrying the Cre transgene is bred with a mouse carrying the floxed gene (F_0 generation). In the progeny (F_1), the floxed gene will be recombined in all Cre-expressing cells. If Cre is driven by a cell-specific promoter, recombination will be restricted to just those cells; if Cre is driven by a universally-expressed promoter, recombination will be universal.

In 1992, two groups (Lakso et al., 1992; Orban et al., 1992) reported the first use of Cre in mice to achieve tissue-specific expression. In 1994, Rajewsky and colleagues (Gu et al., 1994) employed Cre as a conditional gene-targeting tool to circumvent the pleiotropic embryonic lethality of the same null mutation. Tissue-specific Cre-mediated conditional gene inactivation has enabled investigators to address questions that would be otherwise intractable in global knockouts (Lewandoski, 2001). However, as mentioned, to best simulate treatment with a drug, which permeates the entire body, inactivation of the target gene should take place in every tissue type — and thus Cre expression should be driven by a universally-expressed promoter such as the hybrid chicken beta-actin promoter and cytomegalovirus enhancer (CAG) promoter. This promoter was dramatically shown to drive expression of enhanced green fluorescent protein (EGFP) in virtually every cell type to produce green mice (Okabe et al., 1997) (**Figure 2**).

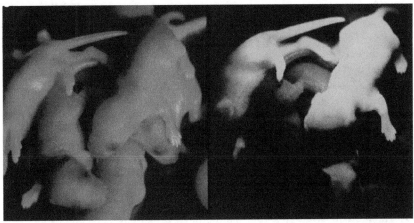

Fig. 2. The transgenic CAG promoter drives expression universally. Five mouse pups are seen under normal light (left); under blue light excitation (right), two of the pups fluoresce green as a result of expression of the ubiquitous CAG promoter that drives EGFP expression in all cell types (in the mice, only red blood cells and hair are not green) (From: Okabe et al., 1997, with permission).

2.1 Modified, ligand-activated CreERT enables temporal control over target gene modulation

To achieve temporal control of Cre recombination, Chambon and colleagues (Feil et al., 1996; Metzger & Chambon, 2001; Metzger et al., 1995) created a ligand-dependent version of Cre, the chimeric protein CreERT, which mediates recombination only in the presence of the drug tamoxifen or its derivatives. In CreERT, Cre is fused to the mutated ligand-binding domain of the estrogen receptor, which recognizes tamoxifen and 4OH-tamoxifen, but not endogenous estrogen (**Figure 3a**). As a steroid receptor of the nuclear receptor family, the estrogen receptor in its inactive form is restricted to the cytoplasm via association with chaperone proteins (Giguère, 2003). As with estrogen activation of the native steroid receptor, tamoxifen releases CreERT from chaperone proteins, enabling the recombinase to diffuse into the nucleus to mediate site-specific recombination (**Figure 3b**). Consequently, target gene-inactivation is temporally controlled and tamoxifen-dependent, as CreERT remains in the cytoplasm until tamoxifen-administration, and returns to the cytoplasm once tamoxifen is no longer in the system.

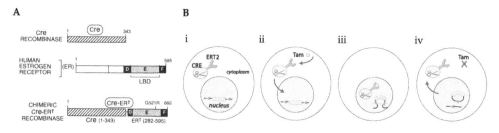

Fig. 3. Temporally controlled, ligand-dependent Cre-lox recombination. A. A mutated version (Gly521→Arg) of the estrogen receptor ligand binding domain (LBD) that recognizes tamoxifen but not estrogen was fused to the Cre protein, resulting in the chimeric protein CreERT (From Metzger & Chambon, 2001, with permission). B. In the absence of tamoxifen or derivatives, the location of CreERT is restricted to the cytoplasm by association with chaperone proteins (i). When engaged by its high-affinity, high-specificity ligand tamoxifen, CreERT is released from the chaperone proteins and diffuses into the nucleus (ii), only then allowing Cre access to recombine genomic DNA irreversibly (iii & iv). After tamoxifen clearance, CreERT will again become sequestered in the cytoplasm (iv).

An enhanced version, CreERT2, is now generally used as it has about a 4-fold greater induction efficiency over CreERT (Indra et al., 1999; Lewandoski, 2001 citations 112-115). For some transgene combinations, there may be some recombination in the absence of tamoxifen (**Figure 4**) (Hayashi, 2002), so evaluation of the magnitude of pre-tamoxifen recombination will therefore be a necessary control. Several ubiquitous inducible Cre lines are available (**Table 1**). An alternate strategy employs a modified progesterone receptor that is activated by RU486 (Kellendonk et al., 1999).

Cre line	Strain name	Stock Number
CagCreERT1	B6.Cg-Tg(CAG-cre/Esr1*)5Amc/J	004682
RosaCreERT2	B6.129-Gt(ROSA)26Sortm1(cre/ERT2)Tyj/J	008463
UBC-CreERT2	B6.Cg-Tg(UBC-cre/ERT2)1Ejb/J	008085

Table 1. Ubiquitously expressed inducible Cre lines. Mice are readily available (jaxmice.jax.org).

Until recently, mice with floxed alleles were generated in individual laboratories and the range of commercially available lines of mice with floxed alleles was limited. Now, floxed mice are being made systematically through a multinational consortium, the Knockout Mouse Project (www.komp.org) (Skarnes et al., 2011). The goal of KOMP is to produce conditional alleles of all expressed mouse genes. So far, 9,000 floxed alleles are or will soon be available, and floxed alleles for the remainder of mouse genes should be accessible in the near term. This comprehensive resource provides the basis for systematic target evaluation using genetic pharmacotherapy.

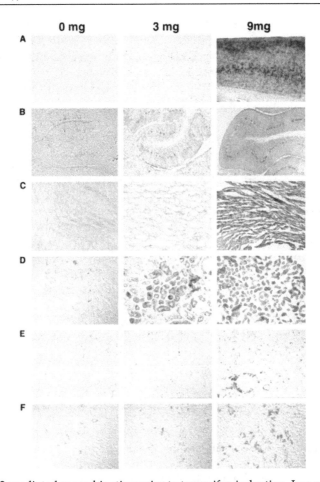

Fig. 4. CreERT2-mediated recombination prior to tamoxifen induction. In a small percentage of cells, recombination occurs in (A) cerebral cortex, (B) cerebellum, (C) heart, (D) kidney, (E) lung, and (F) liver in the absence of tamoxifen (left-most column), as shown by β-galactosidase expression, with the CagCreERT2 mouse line. After tamoxifen (doses shown on top) there is a massive induction of expression (From: Hayashi, 2002, with permission).

3. Comparability to target-specific drugs, with advantages and limitations

Using inducible Cre-lox recombination to inhibit target gene expression offers comparability to, as well as many advantages over, ligand-based inhibition for proof-of-concept studies. Comparable to pharmacologic treatment, genetic pharmacotherapy enables control over the degree of target modulation, analogous to adjustments in drug dose, to assess dose-response; and it also mimics the global, organism-wide action of drug intervention, which enables assessment of possible side effects due to pleiotropic target expression. The strategy's advantages include preclusion of off-target effects via perfect target-specificity, and access to targets in the CNS via permeation of the blood-brain-barrier, which stymies the evaluation of many drug candidates for CNS disorders. There are limitations; these include relative difficulty in targeting splice variants (protein isoforms from the same gene), as the strategy works at the DNA level, and an inability to capture the subtleties of drug action at targets that exhibit functional heterogeneity, i.e. differential structural conformations, drug affinities, and function of a single gene product. We examine each of these points in further illustration below.

3.1 Relative change induced in target-protein function is commensurate to agonism and antagonism

Often, in order to evoke a response in the host cell system, a drug need occupy only a fraction of the total receptors available—a function of both the drug's affinity and the intrinsic ability of the drug-receptor interaction to induce cellular change. This causes the dose-response curve to shift to the left of the receptor occupancy curve, so that a drug dose that elicits maximal tissue response may cause only partial occupation of the available receptors (**Figure 5**).

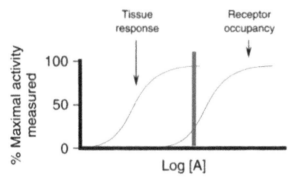

Fig. 5. Maximal tissue response at sub-maximal receptor occupancy. Based on efficacy, drug doses generally need to activate only a fraction of the total available receptors to induce a maximal tissue response. In this illustration, the drug dose that induces maximal tissue response (red line) activates only a fraction of the total available receptors. (Modified from: Ross & Kenakin, 2001, with permission from the McGraw-Hill Companies, Inc.)

For example, opiate agonists etorphine and sufentanil have significant analgesic activity at very low receptor occupancy — approximately 2% at the ED_{50} (Rosenbaum et al., 1984); and in another example, only 22% receptor occupancy is needed for half-maximal stimulation by PEG-TPOm, a mimetic peptide agonist in development for protection against chemotherapy-induced thrombocytopenia (loss of blood platelets) (Samtani et al., 2009). The antipsychotic dopamine D2 receptor antagonist olanzapine achieves optimal clinical efficacy at about 60% receptor occupancy (Mamo et al., 2007).

Similarly, genetic pharmacotherapy need not produce full target inhibition in order to elicit a response. Quantitative gradation in target protein expression (in analogy to a drug dose range) can be controlled by floxing one or both alleles of the gene of interest, and by tamoxifen dose (**Figure 6**) and frequency of administration; in adult mice, tamoxifen is generally administered once daily for 5 days to achieve full recombination. Varying tamoxifen dosing can then mimic the range of drug action.

While the Cre-lox strategy can also be used to simulate agonism, as discussed in later sections, we focus mainly on its application to simulate target antagonism, as the majority of drugs are inhibitors (Copeland et al., 2007; Li et al., 2007) and the accessibility of both ubiquitous CreERT2 mice and the floxed target of choice should now enable systematic *in vivo* target evaluation.

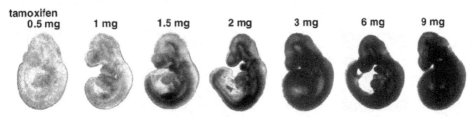

| tamoxifen 0.5 mg | 1 mg | 1.5 mg | 2 mg | 3 mg | 6 mg | 9 mg |

Fig. 6. Tamoxifen dose-dependent recombination in embryos with CreERT driven by a universally expressed promoter. Although Cre-mediated gene modulation is irreversible, "dosing" as a percentage of cells undergoing recombination can still be controlled. Whole-mount transgenic embryos were assayed 9.5 days post-coitum for activity of target gene, β-galactosidase, whose expression had been induced by tamoxifen at the indicated doses (per 40 kg mouse weight) 24 hours prior via intraperitoneal injection of the pregnant dam. (From: Hayashi, 2002, with permission).

To evaluate potential therapeutic efficacy of target modulation, biomarkers or surrogate endpoints specific to the disease model can be used as a response measure — for example, the lowering of blood glucose for genetic pharmacotherapy interventions in diabetes models, LDL cholesterol levels in dyslipidemia models, or PET imaging of ligand binding in CNS models.

3.2 Ubiquitously expressed effector simulates organism-wide pharmacologic actions
In this gene expression modulation system, the effector protein CreERT2 controls the expression of the target gene (for the candidate drug target). In order to achieve the closest simulation of a pharmacologic agent, which has organism-wide effects, it is paramount that a ubiquitously expressed locus such as Rosa26 (Soriano, 1999; Ventura et al., 2007) be used to drive the effector protein expression (**Table 1**). This way it is possible to assess the phenotypic consequences of pleiotropy occurring in targets — that is, the side effects arising from inhibiting a gene product that participates in multiple signaling or metabolic pathways or in different tissues (for further discussion of the relevance of pleiotropies to pharmacotherapy, see Hodgkin, 1998; Searls, 2003). While small interfering RNA (siRNA) has been used extensively for controlled gene inhibition in proof-of-concept studies, siRNA is not drug-like, as it must be delivered to the tissue of interest (Davidson & McCray, 2011).

3.3 Superiority over pharmacologics: preclusion of off-target effects via perfect target-specificity
Since Paul Ehrlich, drug design has aspired to the ideal of "magic bullet" drugs that seek out only "enemy targets" involved in pathology while leaving the body unharmed (Parascandola, 1981). Lack of target specificity not only severely limits the use of small molecules as therapeutics — for example, the clinical use of anti-Parkinsonian drugs pergolide and cabergoline has been greatly limited because their off-target effects cause

valvular heart disease (Keiser et al., 2009) — but also restricts their use as experimental tools in proof-of-concept evaluation (Peterson, 2008). Although promiscuous targeting and multi-receptor activity do produce therapeutic benefits when single-receptor action does not — for example, in the case of statins and psychotropic medications (Keiser et al., 2009; Peterson, 2008) — it is nonetheless preferable that well-defined functional outcomes be understood through well-delineated biochemical actions. Even a drug with high specificity that achieves a desirable outcome in an animal model or clinically still cannot be concluded to work only via the pathway assumed. Genetic pharmacotherapy, on the other hand, enables demonstration of precise, controlled causality in *in vivo* studies.

This is not to say that benefits of polypharmacy cannot be addressed with genetic pharmacotherapy; indeed, the synergy of inhibiting multiple targets simultaneously could be assessed in mice with multiple floxed alleles or by combining genetic pharmacotherapy with traditional pharmacotherapy. It may be impractical to translate findings from such an experiment into a ligand that accomplishes the same synergistic inhibition, but it would enable investigators to parse precisely which targets mediate the desired results, and could guide drug optimization efforts.

Along these lines, genetic pharmacotherapy raises the possibility of validating previously established targets. For example, every antipsychotic drug approved so far has dopamine D2 receptor-blocking activity based on the presumed mode of action of first-generation antipsychotics, which was an entirely serendipitous discovery. However, it likely that their therapeutic efficacy involves interaction with other targets; for instance, antipsychotics inhibit *KCNH2*, a recently described potassium channel, found to be overexpressed in the brains of patients with schizophrenia (Huffaker et al., 2009). The authors state:

> "Whereas D2 receptor affinity is thought to account for the therapeutic effects of antipsychotics, KCNH2 binding is responsible at least for side effects such as altered QT interval or even sudden cardiac failure. Given that KCNH2 controls neuronal excitability and firing patterns, could the therapeutic effects of antipsychotic drugs also be related to their affinities for the brain-specific isoforms of KCNH2? (Huffaker et al., 2009)"

With the present lack of specific KCNH2 ligands, genetic pharmacotherapy could enable further dissection of this possibility and resolve the conceptual justifications guiding the development of compounds with similarly intended actions, pharmacologic or therapeutic.

3.4 Specific advantages with regard to CNS targets

Genetic pharmacotherapy offers particular advantages for proof-of-concept studies for CNS disorders. Such studies face not only the obstacle of designing high-affinity, high-specificity ligands, as in evaluation of targets in other tissues, but also the blood-brain barrier — the superfine filter composed of endothelial cells lining brain capillaries and astrocytes — that either blocks or actively transports out more than 98% of candidate drugs (Miller, 2002). Genetic pharmacotherapy circumvents this obstacle because tamoxifen permeates the blood-brain barrier freely.

3.5 Limitations of achieving target inhibition via DNA modification

While drugs can distinguish between different protein isoforms arising from RNA splice variants (Thompson et al., 2011) that may have different anatomical and functional specificities (Huffaker et al., 2009), genetic pharmacotherapy cannot make such a distinction easily, as target inhibition is mediated via changes at the DNA level. Similarly, a drug may interact differentially with receptors exhibiting functional heterogeneity — e.g. a receptor with distinct allosteric conformations and signaling complexes, varying by anatomical distribution (Mailman, 2007; Mailman & Murthy, 2010) — a subtlety less amenable to simulation with genetic pharmacotherapy but achievable in some cases with pharmacology. The D2 dopamine receptor provides a classic example: agonist stimulation of presynaptic D2 dopamine autoreceptors diminishes dopamine synthesis and release, which may achieve a dopamine antagonist-like effect post-synaptically via decreased dopamine neurotransmission -- whereas preferential agonism of post-synaptic D2 dopamine receptors would achieve the opposite effect. Selective targeting of distinct cell-type D2 receptors cannot be achieved with a universal CreERT line, but the D2 receptor partial agonist aripiprazole appears to exhibit such functional selectivity. Nevertheless, a judiciously chosen tissue-specific inducible CreERT2 strategy may allow such issues to be addressed with better precision than with pharmacology. For instance, presynaptic dopamine D2 receptors have been selectively targeted using a DAT-Cre driver (Bello et al., 2011), and DAT-CreERT2 mice have been reported (Engblom et al., 2008), so that such changes could be induced in adulthood to model an autoreceptor selective dopamine D2 receptor antagonist.

4. Evolution of genetic pharmacotherapy

Genetic pharmacotherapy builds on molecular developments of the last two decades. Below we describe seminal applications of aspects of the genetic pharmacotherapy strategy, and, in certain instances, the molecular entities with actions mirroring the corresponding genetic intervention. Where we wish to build on these foundations is in illustrating the feasibility and advantages of applying this concept — specifically, by employing inducible Cre-lox technology — to evaluate new potential therapeutic drug targets systematically, particularly in the CNS, a possibility that has not yet been articulated until now.

4.1 Genetic blockade *in lieu* or absence of pharmacologic blockade

The potential advantages of using genetic blockade in place of a pharmacologic blockade for CNS studies were described in 1996 in studies reporting the first transgenic expression of Cre in the mouse nervous system (Tsien et al., 1996):

> "Studies of … mechanisms underlying … vertebrate animal [behavior] have traditionally been carried out using pharmacological blockades…. gene knockouts provide an alternative means. While the two methods are complementary, genetic deletion is generally superior to pharmacological blockade with respect to molecular and anatomical specificities and animal-to-animal reproducibility. For instance, while many antagonists cannot distinguish receptor isoforms, genetic blockade can make that distinction. Likewise… a genetic blockade can be highly confined and reproducible."

The juxtaposition of genetic and pharmacologic blockade, in this instance, pertains to their relative merits as experimental tools for addressing questions regarding memory formation as opposed to new therapeutic targets. In a related, concurrent study, the tetracycline transactivator system (described below) was used for regional and temporal control over calcium-calmodulin-dependent kinase II (CamKII) expression to demonstrate the requirement of CamKII for both implicit and explicit memory formation (Mayford et al., 1996).

4.1.1 Tetracycline-regulatable gene expression

The tetracycline transactivator system (Gossen & Bujard, 1992) offers another ligand-controlled gene expression system, in which the targeted gene is turned off or on by the administration of tetracycline or (more commonly) doxycycline (**Figure 7a**). In this system, the *E. coli*-derived tetracycline-controlled transactivator (tTA) drives target-gene transcription by binding to a modified *tet* operator (*tet*O) sequence, and this activity can be diminished and switched off depending on varying concentrations of doxycycline. This strategy is adapted from the *E. coli* tetracycline-resistance operon, in which transcription of tetracycline resistance-mediating genes is negatively regulated by the tetracycline repressor (*tet*R). The presence of tetracycline causes the dissociation of *tet*R from the promoter region of the operon and enables transcription of resistance genes. In contrast, as just mentioned, the modified transactivator tTA, based on *tet*R, *stimulates* (as opposed to repressing) transcription when bound to minimal promoters fused to *tet*O sequences, and the presence of low concentrations of tetracycline (<100 nM) or doxycycline prevents the binding of tTA to the tetO sequences and thereby halts transcription. In the modified tet-on version of this system (Kistner et al., 1996), doxycycline turns on target gene expression via a reverse tTA (rtTA). In this case, rtTA will bind tetO to activate transcription only in the presence of doxycycline (**Figure 7b**).

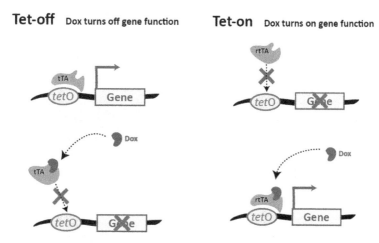

Fig. 7. Tetracycline transactivator (tTA)-controlled gene expression. (a) In tet-off gene regulation, the effector protein tTA binds to the *tet*O promoter, which activates transcription of the target gene. Upon the administration of doxycycline, tTA changes conformation and ceases to activate the target gene's transcription. (b) In the tet-on system, a modified *reverse* tTA (rtTA) binds *tet*O only in the presence of doxycycline.

While the tet-regulatable strategy is appealing for the reversibility of target modulation (with the addition or removal of doxycycline administration) in inhibition studies, it is impossible to produce a silent mutation in the target gene, such as the introduction of loxP sites. In order to control the gene of interest, the *tet*O promoter must be substituted for the native promoter on one allele of the target gene, and the native promoter on the other allele, in turn, used to drive tTA. A study employed this strategy (**Figure 8**) to examine the role of the dopamine transporter (DAT) in scaling learning (Cagniard et al., 2006).

In this tandem design, tissue specificity of target gene expression is maintained, but pre-doxycycline expression levels vary considerably; this is problematic for genetic pharmacotherapy because target gene function should be at basal levels prior to induction. In the strategy illustrated in **Figure 8**, the mutant mice expressed modestly reduced levels of DAT, and it took several weeks of doxycycline administration to achieve significant suppression of DAT expression (Cagniard et al., 2006). In another study examining the role of potassium SK3 channels, SK3 expression was several fold higher than control, and was suppressed with doxycycline (Bond et al., 2000).

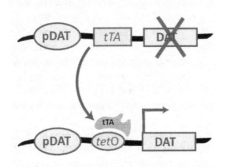

Fig. 8. Target inhibition with tet-off system. For doxycycline-induced knockdown of the targeted dopamine transporter (DAT) function, tTA is expressed under the control of the DAT promoter pDAT on one allele, abrogating DAT expression at that locus; endogenous DAT expression at the other allele is also disrupted by placement of the *tet*O promoter ahead of the gene — but in cells with endogenous pDAT promoter activity driving tTA expression, DAT will be expressed via the *tet*O promoter. Thus tissue specificity of target expression is maintained. Doxycycline then blocks tTA action and so inhibits all DAT expression.

Though less ideal for systematic target evaluation when compared to CreERT2, the tetracycline-transactivator system has nevertheless been particularly powerful in modeling a disease state and subsequently assaying the proof-of-concept of its reversibility via doxycycline administration. In a landmark paper, Yamamoto and colleagues (2000) created a mouse model of Huntington's disease (HD) by *tet*O-driven, striatum-restricted expression of a pathogenic version of the Huntingtin protein. By 4 weeks of age, the mice began to exhibit choreic movements and dystonia, and by 8 weeks showed striatal Huntingtin aggregates — both hallmarks of HD. HD is progressive, without a specific treatment or cure, and prior to this study was assumed to be inexorable in its course. However, abolishing the expression of mutant Huntingtin by doxycycline administration in symptomatic mice not only halted but also *reversed* the accumulation of protein aggregates and progressive motor decline. Although developing a pharmacologic intervention for HD has yet to be achieved, this study demonstrated that blocking expression of pathogenic Huntingtin in symptomatic subjects reversed manifestations of the disease, and indeed could be viewed as having achieved *a cure*. This proof-of-concept clearly motivates a search for drugs that would reverse or prevent Huntingtin protein aggregate formation.

Kellendonk and colleagues (2006) used the tetracycline-transactivator system to address the possibility of reversing schizophrenia-like abnormalities induced by dopamine D2 receptor overexpression (D2OE) in the striatum. Imaging studies have shown that dopamine transmission is increased in patients with schizophrenia, involving both increased dopamine release and increased dopamine D2 receptor binding (Guillin et al., 2007). The D2OE mice, in which tTA drove striatally restricted expression of an extra human D2R allele, exhibited elevated receptor binding capacity — 15% higher than control littermates. The pivotal finding was that dopamine dysfunction — previously thought only to account for the positive symptoms, such as hallucinations and delusions — could be causally linked to cognitive deficits (Simpson et al., 2010). D2OE mice showed altered dopamine transmission in the prefrontal cortex as well as selective cognitive impairment in working memory tasks, a prefrontal cortex-dependent process, without more general cognitive deficits — similar to cognitive impairments in patients with schizophrenia. Administering doxycycline to reverse the D2OE did not reverse the working memory impairment, suggesting that the cognitive deficits in these mice arose not from continued D2OE but as a consequence of D2OE during development. Whether D2OE occurs prior to the onset of schizophrenia in patients is not known; however, dopamine release is increased (Howes et al., 2008), so there is clear evidence for increased dopamine transmission prior to the onset of schizophrenic symptoms. The earlier consequences of increased dopamine transmission in the D2OE mice are consistent with the well-recognized inability of dopamine D2 receptor antagonists to ameliorate cognitive impairments. It must also be noted that while genetic blockade of transgene expression accomplished down-regulation of D2 receptor overexpression, it did not mimic actual D2 receptor antagonist pharmacotherapy fully, as doxycycline inhibited only the transgenic D2 receptors while D2 antagonists would block both the transgenic as well as native D2 receptors. In these studies, the tetracycline-transactivator system was used to model a disease, and subsequently doxycycline administration was used to turn off pathogenic protein expression to establish causality between protein and disease. In genetic pharmacotherapy studies, introduction of an extra tet-regulatable allele could be used to test the effects of increasing target expression, mimicking the actions of a target agonist. One benefit of this strategy, as mentioned, is reversibility of the target modulation; however, the transgenic mice would need to be engineered on a per-target basis, as there is no repository analogous to KOMP for tet-regulatable alleles. Using the tet-off system in inhibition studies, as in the DAT study, disadvantageously requires engineering two transgenic mice (for both the *tet*O and tTA alleles).

4.2 Genetic blockade techniques beyond inducible Cre and tTA

Genetic blockade as a proof-of-concept tool has also been used in a number of oncogenic signaling pathway studies. Although the blockade in the following two examples was accomplished via methods difficult to translate to other druggable targets, the studies successfully established a therapeutic proof-of-concept via genetic means in the absence of a high-specificity ligand against the endogenous target. In one study, a silent mutation engineered into an oncogenic kinase allowed for its selective inhibition, whereas kinase inhibitor non-specificity had previously deterred such an investigation (Fan et al., 2002). In a second study, tumorigenic expression of an endocrine receptor was suppressed by a truncated version of the same receptor (delivered via an adenovirus) that acted as a dominant-negative inhibitor (Min et al., 2003). In both cases, the subsequently developed pharmacologic inhibitors produced the same effect as the genetic blockade, corroborating the parallel between genetic and pharmacologic target blockade.

4.2.1 Engineering a kinase for selective inhibition to determine its role in oncogenic signaling

To overcome the lack of specific kinase inhibitors, Fan and colleagues engineered a silent mutation into a target kinase gene that allowed selective inhibition while retaining kinase activity prior to administration of the mutant kinase-specific antagonist, NaPP1 (Fan et al., 2002). Mice subcutaneously injected with cancer cells containing endogenous or NaPP1-sensitized versions of the epithelial growth factor receptor (EGFP) oncogene v-erbB grew tumors of similar size and with similar latencies – but the inhibitor NaPP1 suppressed growth only in tumors with the sensitized allele (**Figure 9**).

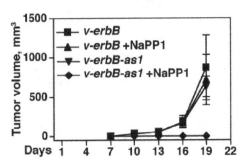

Fig. 9. Chemical genetic blockade in a proof-of-concept study. Assay of tumor growth inhibition in nude mice injected with *v-erbB*- or *v-erbB-as1*-transformed cells. NaPP1 blocks tumor growth only in the mice with the mutagenized *v-erbB-as1* allele that renders the kinase susceptible to selective inhibition by NaPP1 (From: Fan et al., 2002, with permission).

Fan and colleagues (2002) concluded that selective inhibitors of EGFR may effectively arrest cancer cell proliferation at a favorable therapeutic index, as basal signaling in normal cells is unlikely to be affected. Although inhibitors selective for the ErbB EGFR were not available at the time of this chemical-genetic blockade study, genetically engineering inhibitor sensitivity demonstrated the target's proof-of-concept. This incentivized further efforts to develop ligands specific for EGFR subtypes such as ErbB. Indeed, initial marketing of Gefitinib, an EGFR tyrosine kinase inhibitor, was approved in 2003 for patients with non-small cell lung cancer, and Erlotinib, another EGFR tyrosine kinase inhibitor, was approved for the same indication in 2004 and for pancreatic cancer in 2005 (National Cancer Institute Online Drug Information, Pao, 2005).

4.2.2 Virally delivered truncated IGF-I receptor as dominant-negative inhibitor of tumorigenesis

Like EGFR, the insulin-like growth factor I receptor (IGF-Ir) is a mitotic growth factor that stimulates cell growth and is implicated in tumorigenesis (Prager et al., 1994). In certain tumors, IGF-Ir appears to be essential for both malignant transformation and maintenance of the malignant state (Baserga, 1995; Sell et al., 1993). Additionally, initial studies indicated potential tumor selectivity in targeting IGF-Ir for therapeutic applications: reduction of IGF-Ir function induced apoptosis in tumor cells but produced only growth arrest in untransformed cells; and IGF-Ir knockout mice are viable, indicating it is not indispensable for relatively normal development (Min et al., 2003). Prior to the availability of selective ligands, blocking receptor function was accomplished by introducing into tumor cells a recombinant, truncated version of the IGF-Ir with a deleted intracellular tyrosine kinase domain, enabling non-functional heterodimerization. Genetic blockade via dominant-negative receptor expression prevented the formation of sarcomas in nude mice (Prager et al., 1994) and was successful in treating lung, colorectal, and pancreatic xenograft models (Min et al., 2003). Since then, a number of small-molecule IGF-Ir inhibitors have been discovered, with anti-neoplastic action in a wide range of cancers (Carboni et al., 2009; Flanigan et al., 2010; García-Echeverría et al., 2004; He et al., 2010; Iwasa et al., 2009; Kurio et al., 2011), including several that have now moved into clinical trials (Carboni et al., 2009; Iwasa et al., 2009).

4.3 Genetic pharmacotherapy simulates ligand-mediated restoration of p53 anti-tumor activity

Ventura and colleagues did the study — outside the CNS — that most closely embodies our vision of genetic pharmacotherapy (Ventura et al., 2007). They restored function of the transcription factor p53, which has tumor suppressor activity, via a global inducible Cre strategy. p53 was shown in 1991 to be the most frequently inactivated protein in human cancer (Hollstein et al., 1991) so its pathway has been of longstanding interest, and has been the subject of molecular therapeutic development efforts (Vassilev, 2004). Pharmacological restoration of p53 protein function to achieve tumor regression was achieved indirectly by disrupting its interaction with its suppressor protein, MDM2. Indeed, a series of small molecules named Nutlins were discovered that are active in the mid-nanomolar range (Vassilev, 2004).

Ventura and colleagues sought to determine whether rescuing p53 function directly would induce apoptosis and tumor regression. They made p53-LSL mice in which p53 is knocked out due to the insertion of a floxed-Stop (lox-Stop-lox, "LSL") cassette — which stops transcription ahead of the p53 gene — but can be restored by Cre-mediated removal of the cassette. These mice were bred with global ROSA26-CreERT2 mice to produce p53 knockout mice in which tamoxifen could restore p53 function. After irradiating double mutant progeny shortly after birth to accelerate tumor formation, they then showed that tamoxifen treatment of the CreERT2-bearing p53-LSL mice resulted in regression of autochthonous lymphomas and sarcomas, without affecting normal tissues (**Figure 10**).

4.4 Contrasting inducible Cre-lox genetic pharmacotherapy with other modes of genetic blockade

For each of the three targets discussed above for cancer therapy — EGFR, IGF-Ir, and p53 — the drug effects mirror those of the genetic pharmacotherapy intervention, corroborating the technique's comparability as a means of testing a pharmacologic proof-of-concept. Although the Nutlin molecules increase p53 activity indirectly via MDM2 inhibition, and a genetic intervention more directly analogous to the corresponding drug might have targeted a floxed-MDM2 allele, the two studies nonetheless demonstrate the anti-tumor effects (proof-of-concept) of p53-up-regulation (**Figure 11**).

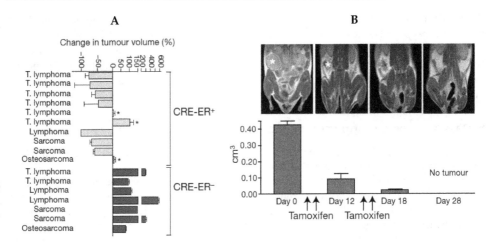

Fig. 10. Genetic pharmacotherapy mediates up-regulation of p53 expression and causes regression of autochthonous sarcomas and lymphomas. A. Tamoxifen administration caused tumor regression in p53-LSL mice expressing tamoxifen-inducible CreERT2, but not in CreERT2-negative p53-LSL mice. B. A series of MRI images (top) shows the regression of an abdominal lymphoma (indicated by the white asterisk) after the administration of tamoxifen. Below, the tumor volume at the time point of each corresponding MRI image. (From: Ventura et al., 2007, with permission)

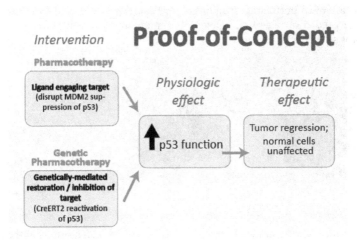

Fig. 11. Parallels in proof-of-concept studies for drug development between ligand-based pharmacotherapy and genetic pharmacotherapy, as exemplified by p53 up-regulation for cancer pharmacotherapy (Vassilev, 2004; Ventura et al., 2007). Both ligand inhibition of MDM2 and tamoxifen-inducible Cre-mediated rescue of homozygous null p53 alleles result in an up-regulation of p53 function that halts tumor cell growth and causes apoptosis, leading to tumor reduction in mice.

While genetically engineering a target for selective inhibition successfully demonstrated the proof-of-concept of EGFR knockdown as cancer therapy — as did expression of a dominant-negative protein to inactivate the endogenous target IGF-Ir — these techniques are highly system-specific and impractical for application to systematic target validation. Inducible Cre-lox recombination technology, on the other hand, can function as a *wild card* enabling ubiquitous modulation of the target of choice.

5. Past and current opportunities for genetic pharmacotherapy applications

A striking example of how genetic pharmacotherapy could have sped up target-validation and substantiated drug discovery efforts is illustrated by dopamine D3 receptor ligand development for the treatment of schizophrenia. Improved treatments that target novel mechanisms implicated in schizophrenia pathophysiology are urgently needed, as current therapies provide little if any alleviation for negative symptoms (anhedonia, social withdrawal) or cognitive symptoms (working memory, attention processing, cognitive flexibility) and furthermore bear a significant side effect profile that contributes to dramatically high patient non-adherence (>74%) (Lieberman et al., 2005). In the 1980s, studies on propsychotic drugs such as amphetamine showed that the drugs elicit maximal dopamine release in the ventral striatum (Di Chiara & Imperato, 1988), whereas antipsychotic extrapyramidal side effects (movement disorders) were thought to arise from interrupting dopamine release in nigrostriatal connections (Grace & Bunney, 1986). It thus became a longstanding pharmacologic goal to block ventral dopaminergic transmission selectively while leaving the dorsal nigrostriatal connections implicated in motor control unaffected in order to achieve a better side effect profile. So, when cloned in 1990, and seen to be distributed just in the ventral striatum (**Figure 12**), the dopamine D3 receptor immediately became a promising drug target for the treatment of schizophrenia (Sokoloff et al., 1990). The prediction was that D3 selective antagonists would prove therapeutic with reduced motor side effects.

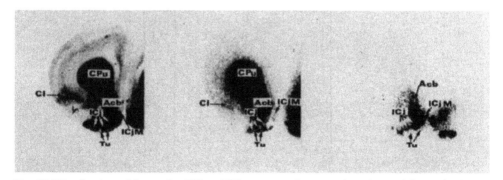

Fig. 12. Distribution of dopamine D2 and D3 receptors in coronal sections of the rat brain. Autoradiographic visualization of the dopamine D2/D3 receptor ligand [125I] iodosulpride binding in a coronal section through the caudate-putamen (CPu) reveals the distribution of dopamine D2 receptors (left). While the distribution of dopamine D2 mRNA revealed by 32P labeled probes (center) matches the iodosulpiride binding, D3 mRNA is localized preferentially in the ventral striatum, principally the nucleus accumbens (Acb), the islands of Calleja (ICj) and the olfactory tubercle (Tu). (From: Sokoloff et al., 1990, with permission).

Although a recently revealed amino acid difference between the highly homologous D2 and D3 receptors will provide new guidance for the design of new D3 receptor-selective ligands together with resolution of the crystal structure (Chien et al., 2010), sufficiently selective ligands are still not available (Lã Ber et al., 2011). Because of the catch-22 that therapeutic efficacy of drug targeting cannot be tested until selective ligands are available, and because the past two decades have yet to yield a sufficiently selective ligand, the proof-of-concept study to demonstrate the therapeutic potential of selective D3 inhibition has yet to be done. Inducing D3 knockdown via inducible-Cre technology in mice modeling schizophrenia endophenotypes could show whether selective dopamine D3 receptor antagonists would be worth pursuing.

5.1 Genetic pharmacotherapy to test proof-of-concept of glutaminase inhibition
While all antipsychotic drugs in clinical use currently target the dopamine system, dysfunction of glutamatergic synaptic transmission has been repeatedly implicated in the pathophysiology of schizophrenia (Javitt, 2010). Schizophrenia appears to involve NMDA-type glutamate receptor hypofunction, as phencyclidine (PCP), ketamine and other NMDA receptor antagonists induce schizophrenia-like symptoms in normals, exacerbate the condition of patients with schizophrenia, and mimic aspects of the disorder in animals (Javitt, 2007; Moghaddam, 2003). However, PCP and its congeners paradoxically induce glutamate release, and overactivate AMPA/kainate-type glutamate receptors (Moghaddam & Adams, 1998), suggesting that tempering release might prove therapeutic. Indeed, mGluR2/3 agonists attenuate both PCP-induced glutamate release and PCP-induced motor stimulation in rodents, and the mGluR2/3 agonist LY214002 has shown significant promise in early clinical trials (Patil et al., 2007). However, therapeutic benefit has yet to be demonstrated in subsequent clinical trials, suggesting that other ways of modulating glutamatergic transmission should be pursued. One promising target is glutaminase, the mitochondrial enzyme that is the rate-limiting step in the recycling of neurotransmitter glutamate from glutamine, that is thought to catalyze the production of the majority of neurotransmitter glutamate (Kvamme et al., 2001). However, there are no known CNS-active glutaminase inhibiters.

Recent clinical studies identify hyperactivity in hippocampal CA1 as being most associated with schizophrenia and predictive in prodromal patients of the transition to diagnosed schizophrenia (Schobel et al., 2009). This builds on a growing body of evidence pointing to hyperactivity in the hippocampus — presumably due to excessive glutamate transmission — as being a primary node in the pathophysiology of the disorder (Lodge & Grace, 2011); hippocampal hyperactivity drives dopamine neuron firing leading to excessive dopamine release and a positive feedback loop that may drive the transition to schizophrenia (Lisman et al., 2010). Interestingly, mice heterozygous for Gls1, the gene encoding glutaminase, exhibit a relative hypoactivity in hippocampal CA1 (Gaisler-Salomon et al., 2009)(**Figure 13**) that is the exact *inverse* of the findings of hyperactivity in hippocampal CA1 in prodromal and diagnosed patients with schizophrenia (Schobel et al., 2009).

Reduced glutaminase expression may therefore confer protection from the pathological processes that engender hippocampal hyperactivity in schizophrenia. Glutaminase inhibition should temper the upstream driving cause of disease symptomatology, rather than block downstream effects such as excessive dopamine release.

Consistent with the therapeutic potential of glutaminase inhibition, Gls1 heterozygous mice showed diminished amphetamine-induced locomotor stimulation and striatal dopamine release (Gaisler-Salomon et al., 2009), two animal-model correlates of positive symptoms in schizophrenia. They showed diminished sensitization to amphetamine (Gaisler-Salomon et al., unpublished) — sensitization is thought to be a key process involved in the progression of schizophrenia (Duncan et al., 1999), and in contrast to patients with schizophrenia, *Gls1* hets showed diminished ketamine-induced frontal cortex activation. The mice showed enhanced latent inhibition, a behavioral measure typically diminished in schizophrenia and enhanced by administration of antipsychotic drugs (Weiner & Arad, 2009). Other measures affected in schizophrenia, including pre-pulse inhibition and working memory, were unaffected. Thus, reduction in *Gls1* function engendered endophenotypic changes suggestive of potential resilience to schizophrenia. Moreover, the global glutaminase deficiency seen in *Gls1* hets had its strongest impact in the hippocampus, suggesting that systemic *Gls1* inhibitors should have a similar focal action. Lacking CNS-active glutaminase inhibiters, genetic pharmacotherapy offers a way to test the therapeutic potential of glutaminase inhibition (Gellman et al., 2011).

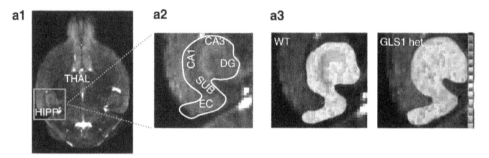

Fig. 13. Cerebral blood volume (CBV) imaging in the hippocampus of *GLs1* het mice. The hippocampal formation (a1, a2) is color-coded in an individual CBV map (a3) such that warmer colors reflect higher CBV values. Regional CBV is fairly uniform across hippocampal subregions in WT mice, but *Gls1* het mice show a selective reduction in the subiculum and CA1. (From: Gaisler-Salomon *et al.* (2009), with permission of the authors).

6. Feasibility and recommendations for systematic use

For disorders with well-defined molecular targets, genetic pharmacotherapy offers a direct way to test the therapeutic potential of inhibiting the target in advance of ligand development. The investigator administers tamoxifen to a disease-modeling mouse carrying both the global-inducible CreERT2 allele and the floxed version of the targeted allele. The resulting DNA recombination event and ensuing change in target expression levels simulates pharmacologic target-modulation. The Knockout Mouse Project (www.komp.org) (Skarnes et al., 2011) now makes available floxed alleles of genes of interest so that the requisite tools are readily or will shortly be available.

While the Cre-ERT2 approach is most directly applicable to antagonism studies, it can also be used for tests of agonism with transgenic mice bearing flox-Stop alleles so that tamoxifen administration would turn on an additional allele or alleles; however, such mice are not widely available. The tTA-tetO system is similarly useful for studies of agonism, which could be most straightforwardly accomplished in transgenic mice bearing the promoter for the target gene driving tTA in tandem with tetO driving the target gene. In contrast, antagonism with tTA-tetO, as noted above, is inherently limited by the inability to design mutant mice in which the target gene is unperturbed. The utility of these approaches is summarized in **Table 2**.

In psychiatric disorders such as schizophrenia, molecular targets are less well defined. Diagnosis remains symptom-based due to lack of specific biomarkers or objective diagnostic tests. Mouse models capture many dimensions of the disorder but cannot be said to be models of the disorder (Arguello & Gogos, 2006; Nestler & Hyman, 2010). As such, for psychiatric disorders, the search for therapeutics is conducted in two stages. In the first stage, recognized behavioral dimensions are evaluated for desired effects of target modulation. For schizophrenia, these dimensions include reduction in correlates of positive symptoms (Carpenter & Koenig, 2008) and negative symptoms (O'Tuathaigh et al., 2010). In the second stage, a mouse model with construct validity — that is, a mouse carrying a mutation known to be implicated in the disease state, or that has been exposed to exogenous agents known to elicit the disorder — is subjected to the same genetic pharmacotherapy and phenomenological assays. Many genetic mouse models have been developed for schizophrenia based on genetic mutations that have been associated with the disorder, both constitutive (Carpenter & Koenig, 2008) and inducible (Pletnikov, 2009). Models based on exogenous agents include *in utero* challenges (Lodge & Grace, 2009), perinatal lesions (Tseng et al., 2009) and drug-induced states (Bickel & Javitt, 2009; Gonzalez-Maeso & Sealfon, 2009).

	CreERT2	tTA-tetO
Antagonism	Ubiquitous CreERT2 :: flox-Target	*(unperturbed control impossible)*
Agonism	Ubiquitous CreERT2:: flox-Stop-Target	pTarget-tTA :: tetO-Target

Table 2. Mouse genetic strategies for genetic pharmacotherapy. Genetic pharmacotherapy can mimic pharmacotherapy for both inhibition (target antagonism) or stimulation (target agonism). CreERT2 is most practical for inhibition studies as the requisite mouse lines (ubiquitous inducible Cre mice, and komp.com-accessible floxed-target mice) are widely available. tTA-tetO cannot be used for inhibition as it is impossible to make a doxycycline-regulatable line without perturbing control expression. Both CreERT2 and tTA-tetO strategies are suitable for stimulation studies, limited by the need to make the requisite mouse lines.

7. Conclusions

The genetic pharmacotherapy strategy enables testing the therapeutic proof-of-concept of target modulation in the absence of specific ligands. It allows circumvention of the proof-of-concept catch-22 in drug development, where the risk of investing in targets with limited validation often impedes the pursuit of specific ligands that would eventually be validated. It also minimizes the complementary problem of investment in selective ligands that would ultimately fail in clinical proof-of-concept studies (**Figure 14**). The recently announced conditional allele library resource (Skarnes et al., 2011) will facilitate efforts to test multiple targets with the inducible Cre strategy. Druggable targets that are likely to be disease modifying have now been identified (Hajduk et al., 2005; Knox et al., 2011; Zhu et al., 2010). The concept and tools of genetic pharmacotherapy have been well established for some time, but their potential for systematic application to proof-of-concept evaluation for drug development efforts has not been fully appreciated. Genetic pharmacotherapy should prove to be a powerful orthogonal tool (Hardy & Peet, 2004) for drug development.

The lack of investment in truly innovative psychiatric drugs over the past decades underpins the vastly unmet need for better treatments, as the burden of psychiatric illness remains high and current treatments remain ineffective or nonexistent (Brundtland, 2001; Miller, 2010). Critics of psychiatric drug development argue that because the etiology of major mental illnesses remains so poorly understood, adequate treatments cannot be developed (Conn & Roth, 2008). However, applying genetic pharmacotherapy in increasingly sophisticated mouse models of psychiatric disorders promises to make the full mouse genome accessible to drug discovery and so expand greatly the accessibility of molecular targets for pharmacotherapies. We believe that this strategy will expedite the development of innovative new molecular therapies, particularly for CNS disorders.

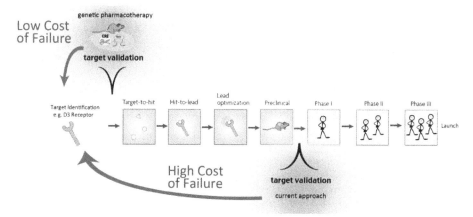

Fig. 14. Role for genetic pharmacotherapy in early stages of the drug development pipeline. Genetic pharmacotherapy (low cost of failure) bypasses ligand development (high cost of failure) in enabling target validation; ligand development (tan shading) can then be implemented for the most promising targets for which proof-of-concept studies demonstrate higher likelihood of success in clinical development (blue shading).

8. Acknowledgements

We are grateful to Anissa Abi-Dargham, Peter Balsam, Laura Bradley, Jay Gingrich, René Hen, Jonathan Javitch, Daniel Javitt, Christoph Kellendonk, Jerry Kokoshka, Jeffrey Lieberman, Holly Moore, Scott Schobel, Scott Small and members of our laboratory for their input and advice on the development of the Genetic Pharmacotherapy strategy. Our research on glutaminase deficient mice is supported by Lieber Center for Schizophrenia Research and Treatment, NIMH Silvio O. Conte Center for Schizophrenia Research (P50 MH066171), and R01 MH087758.

9. References

Arguello, P.A. and Gogos, J.A. (2006) Modeling madness in mice: one piece at a time. *Neuron*, Vol. 52, No. 1, pp. 179-196

Baserga, R. (1995) The insulin-like growth factor I receptor: a key to tumor growth? *Cancer Res.*, Vol. 55, No. 2, pp. 249-252

Bello, E.P., Mateo, Y., Gelman, D.M., Noaín, D., Shin, J.H., Low, M.J., Alvarez, V.A., Lovinger, D.M. and Rubinstein, M. (2011) Cocaine supersensitivity and enhanced motivation for reward in mice lacking dopamine D2 autoreceptors. *Nat. Neurosci.*, Vol. 14, No. 8, pp. 1033-1038

Bickel, S. and Javitt, D. (2009) Neurophysiological and neurochemical animal models of schizophrenia: focus on glutamate. *Behav. Brain Res.*, Vol. 204, No. 2, pp. 352-362

Bond, C.T., Sprengel, R., Bissonnette, J.M., Kaufmann, W.A., Pribnow, D., Neelands, T., Storck, T., Baetscher, M., Jerecic, J., Maylie, J., Knaus, H.G., Seeburg, P.H. and Adelman, J.P. (2000) Respiration and parturition affected by conditional overexpression of the Ca2+-activated K+ channel subunit, SK3. *Science*, Vol. 289, No. 5486, pp. 1942-1946

Brundtland, G.H. (2001) From the World Health Organization. Mental health: new understanding, new hope. *JAMA*, Vol. 286, No. 19, pp. 2391

Cagniard, B., Beeler, J.A., Britt, J.P., McGehee, D.S., Marinelli, M. and Zhuang, X. (2006) Dopamine scales performance in the absence of new learning. *Neuron*, Vol. 51, No. 5, pp. 541-547

Carboni, J.M., Wittman, M., Yang, Z., Lee, F., Greer, A., Hurlburt, W., Hillerman, S., Cao, C., Cantor, G.H., Dell-John, J., Chen, C., Discenza, L., Menard, K., Li, A., Trainor, G., Vyas, D., Kramer, R., Attar, R.M. and Gottardis, M.M. (2009) BMS-754807, a small molecule inhibitor of insulin-like growth factor-1R/IR. *Molecular Cancer Therapeutics*, Vol. 8, No. 12, pp. 3341-3349

Carpenter, W.T. and Koenig, J. (2008) The evolution of drug development in schizophrenia: past issues and future opportunities. *Neuropsychopharmacology*, Vol. 33, No. 9, pp. 2061-2079

Chien, E.Y.T., Liu, W., Zhao, Q., Katritch, V., Han, G.W., Hanson, M.A., Shi, L., Newman, A.H., Javitch, J.A., Cherezov, V. and Stevens, R.C. (2010) Structure of the human dopamine D3 receptor in complex with a D2/D3 selective antagonist. *Science*, Vol. 330, No. 6007, pp. 1091-1095

Conn, P.J. and Roth, B.L. (2008) Opportunities and Challenges of Psychiatric Drug Discovery: Roles for Scientists in Academic, Industry, and Government Settings. *Neuropsychopharmacology*, Vol. 33, No. 9, pp. 2048-2060

Copeland, R.A., Harpel, M.R. and Tummino, P.J. (2007) Targeting enzyme inhibitors in drug discovery. *Expert Opin Ther Targets*, Vol. 11, No. 7, pp. 967-978

Davidson, B.L. and McCray, P.B. (2011) Current prospects for RNA interference-based therapies. *Nature Publishing Group*, Vol. 12, No. 5, pp. 329-340

Di Chiara, G. and Imperato, A. (1988) Drugs abused by humans preferentially increase synaptic dopamine concentrations in the mesolimbic system of freely moving rats. *PNAS*, Vol. 85, No. 14, pp. 5274-5278

Duncan, G.E., Sheitman, B.B. and Lieberman, J.A. (1999) An integrated view of pathophysiological models of schizophrenia. *Brain Res. Brain Res. Rev.*, Vol. 29, No. 2-3, pp. 250-264

Engblom, D., Bilbao, A., Sanchis-Segura, C., Dahan, L., Perreau-Lenz, S., Balland, B., Parkitna, J.R., Luján, R., Halbout, B., Mameli, M., Parlato, R., Sprengel, R., Lüscher, C., Schütz, G. and Spanagel, R. (2008) Glutamate receptors on dopamine neurons control the persistence of cocaine seeking. *Neuron*, Vol. 59, No. 3, pp. 497-508

Fan, Q.-W., Zhang, C., Shokat, K.M. and Weiss, W.A. (2002) Chemical genetic blockade of transformation reveals dependence on aberrant oncogenic signaling. *Curr. Biol.*, Vol. 12, No. 16, pp. 1386-1394

Feil, R., Brocard, J., Mascrez, B., LeMeur, M., Metzger, D. and Chambon, P. (1996) Ligand-activated site-specific recombination in mice. *PNAS*, Vol. 93, No. 20, pp. 10887-10890

Flanigan, S.A., Pitts, T.M., Eckhardt, S.G., Tentler, J.J., Tan, A.C., Thorburn, A. and Leong, S. (2010) The Insulin-like Growth Factor I Receptor/Insulin Receptor Tyrosine Kinase Inhibitor PQIP Exhibits Enhanced Antitumor Effects in Combination with Chemotherapy Against Colorectal Cancer Models. *Clin. Cancer Res.*, Vol. 16, No. 22, pp. 5436-5446

Gaisler-Salomon, I., Miller, G.M., Chuhma, N., Lee, S., Zhang, H., Ghoddoussi, F., Lewandowski, N., Fairhurst, S., Wang, Y., Conjard-Duplany, A., Masson, J., Balsam, P., Hen, R., Arancio, O., Galloway, M.P., Moore, H.M., Small, S.A. and Rayport, S. (2009) Glutaminase-deficient mice display hippocampal hypoactivity, insensitivity to pro-psychotic drugs and potentiated latent inhibition: relevance to schizophrenia. *Neuropsychopharmacology*, Vol. 34, No. 10, pp. 2305-2322

García-Echeverría, C., Pearson, M.A., Marti, A., Meyer, T., Mestan, J., Zimmermann, J., Gao, J., Brueggen, J., Capraro, H.-G., Cozens, R., Evans, D.B., Fabbro, D., Furet, P., Porta, D.G., Liebetanz, J., Martiny-Baron, G., Ruetz, S. and Hofmann, F. (2004) In vivo antitumor activity of NVP-AEW541-A novel, potent, and selective inhibitor of the IGF-IR kinase. *Cancer Cell*, Vol. 5, No. 3, pp. 231-239

Gellman, C., Mingote, S., Wang, Y., Gaisler-Salomon, I. and Rayport, S. (2011) Genetic pharmacotherapy: A new approach to drug development for schizophrenia. *Advancing Drug Discovery for Schizophrenia, NY Academy of Sciences,* New York, NY, 03/18/11

Giguère, V. (2003) In Bradshaw, R. A. and Dennis, E. A. (eds.), *Handbook of Cell Signaling, Volume 3.* Academic Press, Amsterdam, Vol. 3, pp. 35-38.

Gingrich, J.A. and Hen, R. (2000) The broken mouse: the role of development, plasticity and environment in the interpretation of phenotypic changes in knockout mice. *Curr. Opin. Neurobiol.*, Vol. 10, No. 1, pp. 146-152

Gonzalez-Maeso, J. and Sealfon, S.C. (2009) Psychedelics and schizophrenia. *Trends Neurosci.*, Vol. 32, No. 4, pp. 225-232

Gossen, M. and Bujard, H. (1992) Tight control of gene expression in mammalian cells by tetracycline-responsive promoters. *PNAS*, Vol. 89, No. 12, pp. 5547-5551

Grace, A.A. and Bunney, B.S. (1986) Induction of depolarization block in midbrain dopamine neurons by repeated administration of haloperidol: analysis using in vivo intracellular recording. *J. Pharmacol. Exp. Ther.*, Vol. 238, No. 3, pp. 1092-1100

Gu, H., Marth, J.D., Orban, P.C., Mossmann, H. and Rajewsky, K. (1994) Deletion of a DNA polymerase beta gene segment in T cells using cell type-specific gene targeting. *Science*, Vol. 265, No. 5168, pp. 103-106

Guillin, O., Abi-Dargham, A. and Laruelle, M. (2007) Neurobiology of dopamine in schizophrenia. *Int. Rev. Neurobiol.*, Vol. 78, pp. 1-39

Hajduk, P.J., Huth, J.R. and Tse, C. (2005) Predicting protein druggability. *Drug Discovery Today*, Vol. 10, No. 23-24, pp. 1675-1682

Hardy, L.W. and Peet, N.P. (2004) The multiple orthogonal tools approach to define molecular causation in the validation of druggable targets. *Drug Discovery Today,* Vol. 9, No. 3, pp. 117-126

Hayashi, S. (2002) Efficient Recombination in Diverse Tissues by a Tamoxifen-Inducible Form of Cre: A Tool for Temporally Regulated Gene Activation/Inactivation in the Mouse. *Dev. Biol.*, Vol. 244, No. 2, pp. 305-318

He, Y., Zhang, J., Zheng, J., Du, W., Xiao, H., Liu, W., Li, X., Chen, X., Yang, L. and Huang, S. (2010) The insulin-like growth factor-1 receptor kinase inhibitor, NVP-ADW742, suppresses survival and resistance to chemotherapy in acute myeloid leukemia cells. *Oncol. Res.*, Vol. 19, No. 1, pp. 35-43

Hodgkin, J. (1998) Seven types of pleiotropy. *Int. J. Dev. Biol.*, Vol. 42, No. 3, pp. 501-505

Hollstein, M., Sidransky, D., Vogelstein, B. and Harris, C.C. (1991) p53 mutations in human cancers. *Science*, Vol. 253, No. 5015, pp. 49-53

Howes, O., Montgomery, A., Valli, I., Asselin, M., Murray, R., Grasby, P. and Mcguire, P. (2008) Striatal dopamine dysfunction predates the onset of schizophrenia and is linked to prodromal symptoms and neurocognitive function. *Schizophr. Res.*, Vol. 102, No. 1-3, pp. 30-30

Huffaker, S.J., Chen, J., Nicodemus, K.K., Sambataro, F., Yang, F., Mattay, V., Lipska, B.K., Hyde, T.M., Song, J., Rujescu, D., Giegling, I., Mayilyan, K., Proust, M.J., Soghoyan, A., Caforio, G., Callicott, J.H., Bertolino, A., Meyer-Lindenberg, A., Chang, J., Ji, Y., Egan, M.F., Goldberg, T.E., Kleinman, J.E., Lu, B. and Weinberger, D.R. (2009) A primate-specific, brain isoform of KCNH2 affects cortical physiology, cognition, neuronal repolarization and risk of schizophrenia. *Nat. Med.*, Vol. 15, No. 5, pp. 509-518

Indra, A.K., Warot, X., Brocard, J., Bornert, J.M., Xiao, J.H., Chambon, P. and Metzger, D. (1999) Temporally-controlled site-specific mutagenesis in the basal layer of the epidermis: comparison of the recombinase activity of the tamoxifen-inducible Cre-ER(T) and Cre-ER(T2) recombinases. *Nucleic Acids Res.*, Vol. 27, No. 22, pp. 4324-4327

Iwasa, T., Okamoto, I., Suzuki, M., Hatashita, E., Yamada, Y., Fukuoka, M., Ono, K. and Nakagawa, K. (2009) Inhibition of Insulin-Like Growth Factor 1 Receptor by CP-751,871 Radiosensitizes Non-Small Cell Lung Cancer Cells. *Clin. Cancer Res.*, Vol. 15, No. 16, pp. 5117-5125

Javitt, D.C. (2007) Glutamate and schizophrenia: Phencyclidine, n-methyl-d-aspartate receptors, and dopamine-glutamate interactions. *Int. Rev. Neurobiol.*, Vol. 78, pp. 69-108

Javitt, D.C. (2010) Glutamatergic theories of schizophrenia. *Isr. J. Psychiatry Relat. Sci.*, Vol. 47, No. 1, pp. 4-16

Keiser, M.J., Setola, V., Irwin, J.J., Laggner, C., Abbas, A.I., Hufeisen, S.J., Jensen, N.H., Kuijer, M.B., Matos, R.C., Tran, T.B., Whaley, R., Glennon, R.A., Hert, J., Thomas, K.L.H., Edwards, D.D., Shoichet, B.K. and Roth, B.L. (2009) Predicting new molecular targets for known drugs. *Nature*, Vol. 462, No. 7270, pp. 175-181

Kellendonk, C., Simpson, E.H., Polan, H.J., Malleret, G., Vronskaya, S., Winiger, V., Moore, H. and Kandel, E.R. (2006) Transient and selective overexpression of dopamine D2 receptors in the striatum causes persistent abnormalities in prefrontal cortex functioning. *Neuron*, Vol. 49, No. 4, pp. 603-615

Kellendonk, C., Tronche, F., Casanova, E., Anlag, K., Opherk, C. and Schutz, G. (1999) Inducible site-specific recombination in the brain. *J. Mol. Biol.*, Vol. 285, No. 1, pp. 175-182

Kistner, A., Gossen, M., Zimmermann, F., Jerecic, J., Ullmer, C., Lübbert, H. and Bujard, H. (1996) Doxycycline-mediated quantitative and tissue-specific control of gene expression in transgenic mice. *PNAS*, Vol. 93, No. 20, pp. 10933-10938

Knox, C., Law, V., Jewison, T., Liu, P., Ly, S., Frolkis, A., Pon, A., Banco, K., Mak, C., Neveu, V., Djoumbou, Y., Eisner, R., Guo, A.C. and Wishart, D.S. (2011) DrugBank 3.0: a comprehensive resource for 'omics' research on drugs. *Nucleic Acids Res*, Vol. 39, Database issue, pp. D1035-1041

Kurio, N., Shimo, T., Fukazawa, T., Takaoka, M., Okui, T., Hassan, N.M.M., Honami, T., Hatakeyama, S., Ikeda, M., Naomoto, Y. and Sasaki, A. (2011) Anti-tumor effect in human breast cancer by TAE226, a dual inhibitor for FAK and IGF-IR in vitro and in vivo. *Exp. Cell Res.*, Vol. 317, No. 8, pp. 1134-1146

Kvamme, E., Torgner, I.A. and Roberg, B.A. (2001) Kinetics and localization of brain phosphate activated glutaminase. *J. Neurosci. Res.*, Vol. 66, No. 5, pp. 951-958

Lã Ber, S., Hübner, H., Tschammer, N. and Gmeiner, P. (2011) Recent advances in the search for D3- and D4-selective drugs: probes, models and candidates. *Trends Pharmacol. Sci.*, Vol. 32, No. 3, pp. 148-157

Lakso, M., Sauer, B., Mosinger, B., Jr., Lee, E.J., Manning, R.W., Yu, S.H., Mulder, K.L. and Westphal, H. (1992) Targeted oncogene activation by site-specific recombination in transgenic mice. *PNAS*, Vol. 89, No. 14, pp. 6232-6236

Lewandoski, M. (2001) Conditional control of gene expression in the mouse. *Nature Rev Genet*, Vol. 2, No. 10, pp. 743-755

Li, Q.-X., Tan, P., Ke, N. and Wong-Staal, F. (2007) Ribozyme technology for cancer gene target identification and validation. *Adv. Cancer Res.*, Vol. 96, pp. 103-143

Lieberman, J.A., Stroup, T.S., McEvoy, J.P., Swartz, M.S., Rosenheck, R.A., Perkins, D.O., Keefe, R.S., Davis, S.M., Davis, C.E., Lebowitz, B.D., Severe, J. and Hsiao, J.K. (2005) Effectiveness of antipsychotic drugs in patients with chronic schizophrenia. *N. Engl. J. Med.*, Vol. 353, No. 12, pp. 1209-1223

Lisman, J.E., Pi, H.J., Zhang, Y. and Otmakhova, N.A. (2010) A thalamo-hippocampal-ventral tegmental area loop may produce the positive feedback that underlies the psychotic break in schizophrenia. *Biol. Psychiatry*, Vol. 68, No. 1, pp. 17-24

Lodge, D.J. and Grace, A.A. (2009) Gestational methylazoxymethanol acetate administration: a developmental disruption model of schizophrenia. *Behav. Brain Res.*, Vol. 204, No. 2, pp. 306-312

Lodge, D.J. and Grace, A.A. (2011) Hippocampal dysregulation of dopamine system function and the pathophysiology of schizophrenia. *Trends Pharmacol. Sci.*, Vol. 32, No. 9, pp. 507-513

Mailman. (2007) GPCR functional selectivity has therapeutic impact. *Trends Pharmacol. Sci.*, Vol. 28, No. 8, pp. 390-396

Mailman, R.B. and Murthy, V. (2010) Ligand functional selectivity advances our understanding of drug mechanisms and drug discovery. *Neuropsychopharmacology*, Vol. 35, No. 1, pp. 345-346

Mamo, D., Kapur, S., Keshavan, M., Laruelle, M., Taylor, C.C., Kothare, P.A., Barsoum, P. and McDonnell, D. (2007) D2 Receptor Occupancy of Olanzapine Pamoate Depot Using Positron Emission Tomography: An Open-label Study in Patients with Schizophrenia. *Neuropsychopharmacology*, Vol. 33, No. 2, pp. 298-304

Mayford, M., Bach, M.E., Huang, Y.Y., Wang, L., Hawkins, R.D. and Kandel, E.R. (1996) Control of memory formation through regulated expression of a CaMKII transgene. *Science*, Vol. 274, No. 5293, pp. 1678-1683

Metzger, D. and Chambon, P. (2001) Site- and time-specific gene targeting in the mouse. *Methods*, Vol. 24, No. 1, pp. 71-80

Metzger, D., Clifford, J., Chiba, H. and Chambon, P. (1995) Conditional site-specific recombination in mammalian cells using a ligand-dependent chimeric Cre recombinase. *PNAS*, Vol. 92, No. 15, pp. 6991-6995

Miller, G. (2002), *Science*, Vol. 297, pp. 1116-1118.

Miller, G. (2010), *Science*, Vol. 329, pp. 502-504.

Min, Y., Adachi, Y., Yamamoto, H., Ito, H., Itoh, F., Lee, C.-T., Nadaf, S., Carbone, D.P. and Imai, K. (2003) Genetic blockade of the insulin-like growth factor-I receptor: a promising strategy for human pancreatic cancer. *Cancer Res.*, Vol. 63, No. 19, pp. 6432-6441

Moghaddam, B. (2003) Bringing order to the glutamate chaos in schizophrenia. *Neuron*, Vol. 40, No. 5, pp. 881-884

Moghaddam, B. and Adams, B.W. (1998) Reversal of phencyclidine effects by a group II metabotropic glutamate receptor agonist in rats. *Science*, Vol. 281, No. 5381, pp. 1349-1352

Nagy, A. (2000) Cre recombinase: the universal reagent for genome tailoring. *Genesis*, Vol. 26, No. 2, pp. 99-109

Nestler, E.J. and Hyman, S.E. (2010) Animal models of neuropsychiatric disorders. *Nat. Neurosci.*, Vol. 13, No. 10, pp. 1161-1169

O'Tuathaigh, C., Kirby, B., Moran, P. and Waddington, J. (2010) Mutant Mouse Models: Genotype-Phenotype Relationships to Negative Symptoms in Schizophrenia. *Schizophr. Bull.*, Vol. 36, No. 2, pp. 271-288

Okabe, M., Ikawa, M., Kominami, K., Nakanishi, T. and Nishimune, Y. (1997) 'Green mice' as a source of ubiquitous green cells. *FEBS Lett.*, Vol. 407, No. 3, pp. 313-319

Orban, P.C., Chui, D. and Marth, J.D. (1992) Tissue- and site-specific DNA recombination in transgenic mice. *PNAS*, Vol. 89, No. 15, pp. 6861-6865

Pao, W. (2005) Epidermal Growth Factor Receptor Mutations, Small-Molecule Kinase Inhibitors, and Non-Small-Cell Lung Cancer: Current Knowledge and Future Directions. *J. Clin. Oncol.*, Vol. 23, No. 11, pp. 2556-2568

Parascandola, J. (1981) *The theoretical basis of Paul Ehrlich' chemotherapy.*

Patil, S.T., Zhang, L., Martenyi, F., Lowe, S.L., Jackson, K.A., Andreev, B.V., Avedisova, A.S., Bardenstein, L.M., Gurovich, I.Y., Morozova, M.A., Mosolov, S.N., Neznanov, N.G., Reznik, A.M., Smulevich, A.B., Tochilov, V.A., Johnson, B.G., Monn, J.A. and Schoepp, D.D. (2007) Activation of mGlu2/3 receptors as a new approach to treat schizophrenia: a randomized Phase 2 clinical trial. *Nat. Med.*, Vol. 13, No. 9, pp. 1102-1107

Peterson, R.T. (2008) Chemical biology and the limits of reductionism. *Nat. Chem. Biol.*, Vol. 4, No. 11, pp. 635-638

Pletnikov, M.V. (2009) Inducible and conditional transgenic mouse models of schizophrenia. *Prog. Brain Res.*, Vol. 179, pp. 35-47

Prager, D., Li, H.L., Asa, S. and Melmed, S. (1994) Dominant negative inhibition of tumorigenesis in vivo by human insulin-like growth factor I receptor mutant. *PNAS*, Vol. 91, No. 6, pp. 2181-2185

Rosenbaum, J.S., Holford, N.H. and Sadée, W. (1984) Opiate receptor binding-effect relationship: sufentanil and etorphine produce analgesia at the mu-site with low fractional receptor occupancy. *Brain Res.*, Vol. 291, No. 2, pp. 317-324

Ross, E.M. and Kenakin, T.P. (2001) In Goodman, L. S., Hardman, J. G., Limbird, L. E. and Gilman, A. G. (eds.), *Goodman & Gilman's The Pharmacological Basis of Therapeutics.* 10th ed. McGraw-Hill Medical Pub. Division, New York, pp. 31-43.

Samtani, M.N., Perez-Ruixo, J.J., Brown, K.H., Cerneus, D. and Molloy, C.J. (2009) Pharmacokinetic and pharmacodynamic modeling of pegylated thrombopoietin mimetic peptide (PEG-TPOm) after single intravenous dose administration in healthy subjects. *J Clin Pharmacol*, Vol. 49, No. 3, pp. 336-350

Schobel, S.A., Lewandowski, N.M., Corcoran, C.M., Moore, H., Brown, T., Malaspina, D. and Small, S.A. (2009) Differential targeting of the CA1 subfield of the hippocampal formation by schizophrenia and related psychotic disorders. *Arch. Gen. Psychiatry*, Vol. 66, No. 9, pp. 938-946

Searls, D.B. (2003) Pharmacophylogenomics: genes, evolution and drug targets. *Nat Rev Drug Discov*, Vol. 2, No. 8, pp. 613-623

Sell, C., Rubini, M., Rubin, R., Liu, J.P., Efstratiadis, A. and Baserga, R. (1993) Simian virus 40 large tumor antigen is unable to transform mouse embryonic fibroblasts lacking type 1 insulin-like growth factor receptor. *PNAS*, Vol. 90, No. 23, pp. 11217-11221

Simpson, E.H., Kellendonk, C. and Kandel, E. (2010) A possible role for the striatum in the pathogenesis of the cognitive symptoms of schizophrenia. *Neuron*, Vol. 65, No. 5, pp. 585-596

Skarnes, W.C., Rosen, B., West, A.P., Koutsourakis, M., Bushell, W., Iyer, V., Mujica, A.O., Thomas, M., Harrow, J., Cox, T., Jackson, D., Severin, J., Biggs, P., Fu, J., Nefedov, M., de Jong, P.J., Stewart, A.F. and Bradley, A. (2011) A conditional knockout resource for the genome-wide study of mouse gene function. *Nature*, Vol. 474, No. 7351, pp. 337-342

Sokoloff, P., Giros, B., Martres, M.P., Bouthenet, M.L. and Schwartz, J.C. (1990) Molecular cloning and characterization of a novel dopamine receptor (D3) as a target for neuroleptics. *Nature*, Vol. 347, No. 6289, pp. 146-151

Soriano, P. (1999) Generalized lacZ expression with the ROSA26 Cre reporter strain. *Nat. Genet.*, Vol. 21, No. 1, pp. 70-71

Sternberg, N. and Hamilton, D. (1981) Bacteriophage P1 site-specific recombination. I. Recombination between loxP sites. *J. Mol. Biol.*, Vol. 150, No. 4, pp. 467-486

Thompson, C.H., Kahlig, K.M. and George, A.L. (2011) SCN1A splice variants exhibit divergent sensitivity to commonly used antiepileptic drugs. *Epilepsia*, Vol. 52, No. 5, pp. 1000-1009

Tseng, K.Y., Chambers, R.A. and Lipska, B.K. (2009) The neonatal ventral hippocampal lesion as a heuristic neurodevelopmental model of schizophrenia. *Behav. Brain Res.*, Vol. 204, No. 2, pp. 295-305

Tsien, J.Z., Chen, D.F., Gerber, D., Tom, C., Mercer, E.H., Anderson, D.J., Mayford, M., Kandel, E.R. and Tonegawa, S. (1996) Subregion- and cell type-restricted gene knockout in mouse brain. *Cell*, Vol. 87, No. 7, pp. 1317-1326

Vassilev, L.T. (2004) In vivo activation of the p53 pathway by small-molecule antagonists of MDM2. *Science*, Vol. 303, No. 5659, pp. 844-848

Ventura, A., Kirsch, D.G., McLaughlin, M.E., Tuveson, D.A., Grimm, J., Lintault, L., Newman, J., Reczek, E.E., Weissleder, R. and Jacks, T. (2007) Restoration of p53 function leads to tumour regression in vivo. *Nature*, Vol. 445, No. 7128, pp. 661-665

Weiner, I. and Arad, M. (2009) Using the pharmacology of latent inhibition to model domains of pathology in schizophrenia and their treatment. *Behav. Brain Res.*, Vol. 204, No. 2, pp. 369-386

Yamamoto, A., Lucas, J.J. and Hen, R. (2000) Reversal of neuropathology and motor dysfunction in a conditional model of Huntington's disease. *Cell*, Vol. 101, No. 1, pp. 57-66

Zhu, F., Han, B., Kumar, P., Liu, X., Ma, X., Wei, X., Huang, L., Guo, Y., Han, L., Zheng, C. and Chen, Y. (2010) Update of TTD: Therapeutic Target Database. *Nucleic Acids Res*, Vol. 38, No. Database issue, pp. D787-791

6

Genetically Engineered Mouse Models in Preclinical Anti-Cancer Drug Development

Sergio Y. Alcoser and Melinda G. Hollingshead
Biological Testing Branch, Developmental Therapeutics Program,
National Cancer Institute
USA

1. Introduction

According to the most recent American Cancer Society data, an estimated 569,490 Americans died from cancer in 2010 (American Cancer Society [ACS], 2010). The number of cancer-related deaths recently surpassed those from heart disease in Americans <85 yrs old (Kung et al., 2008). Developing new and more efficacious anti-cancer compounds is a paramount health care priority. At the Developmental Therapeutics Program of the U.S. National Cancer Institute, potential therapeutic agents are typically tested for activity in an *in vitro* 60-tumor cell line screen and subsequently by *in vivo* xenograft studies in rodents (Figure 1). Once selected for additional testing using established criteria (drugability, novelty of structure and/or mechanism of action, potency, cell panel selectivity, etc.), additional studies (pharmaocokinetics, pharmacodynamics, range finding toxicity, formulation, mechanism of action analysis, IND-directed toxicology, etc.) are initiated followed by the progression of a selected few candidate agents into human clinical trials. Efficacious drugs with tolerable toxicity are ushered into early phase clinical trials. However, most of the promising compounds identified in the multi-layered preclinical screenings are not as successful in human patients. Therefore, preclinical models that better predict drug efficacy and toxicity in humans are needed. Differences in drug absorption, distribution, metabolism and elimination (ADME), immune responses and over-interpretation of the preclinical efficacy data may contribute to clinical failures. However, a significant limitation is generating mouse models that histologically, genetically, and behaviorally recapitulate the human disease.

Over the past twenty years, researchers have identified many of the underlying genetic abnormalities that cause certain cancers and have genetically engineered them into mouse models to explore the oncogenic nature of those genes and related pathways. The resulting mouse models generate tumors that may better mimic those seen in humans. It is anticipated that therapeutic compounds which show efficacy and low toxicity in these more human-like genetically engineered mouse (GEM) models will be more successful in clinical trials and lead to increased cancer survivorship. Hundreds of GEM models currently exist that are associated with some form of human tumor development (see the eMICE website). It is well beyond the scope of this manuscript to adequately describe each of them. We instead briefly review some of the ground-breaking GEM models developed in the 1980s and 90s, describe more recent and sophisticated models, highlight some of the advantages and limitations for each, and explore the potential roles of molecular targeted therapies and GEM models in preclinical drug testing. For additional details on each model, we refer the reader to the original articles or prior in-depth reviews. While mice that develop genetically engineered tumors hold much promise, the relatively slow growth rate of these tumors and their low penetrance (regardless of genetics, some mice will not develop tumors during the time constraints of the experiment) makes them ill-suited to replace xenograft models as the primary *in vivo* screening tool. Instead, we envision GEM models as an additional screening mechanism that narrows and optimizes the field of therapeutic compounds before expensive and time-consuming human clinical trials are initiated.

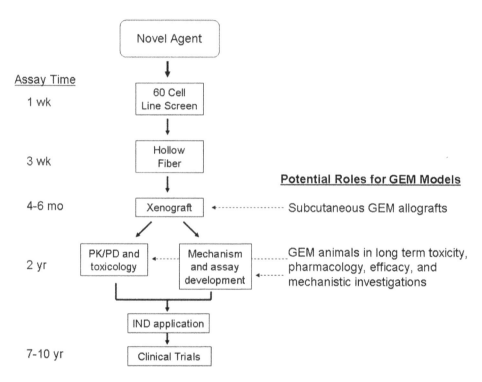

Fig. 1. Where GEMs Can Be Most Useful in the Preclinical Drug Development

Simplistic overview of preclinical drug development procedure in the NCI/DTP. Novel agents are introduced through the 60 Cell Line Screen (reviewed in Monks et al., 1991), which contains 60 human cultured tumor cell lines in a 96-well plate array. If anti-proliferative activity is observed in a number of cell lines, the agent is tested in a Hollow Fiber assay, which measures the anti-proliferative activity in cultured cells grown in hollow polyvinylidene fluoride (PVDF) fibers implanted intraperitoneally and subcutaneously in mice (reviewed in Decker et al., 2004). If active in Hollow Fiber assays, agents are administered to immunodeficient animals that possess human tumors generated from serially passaged human tumor cell lines (xenografts). Tolerable toxicity and activity measurable in xenograft models leads to simultaneous investigations into the agent's

PK/PD, mechanism of action and toxicology. Based on this data, where applicable an IND application is generated for FDA approval to initiate clinical trials. The agents may require further preclinical studies or can be approved for a small scale Phase 0 trial (reviewed in Murgo et al., 2008), or initial Phase I human clinical trials. Assay Time is a best case scenario for a single agent and does not include time for optimization and validation repetitions. PD = pharmacodynamics, PK = pharmacokinetics, GEM = genetically engineered mouse, IND = Investigational New Drug

2. Background: *in vivo* drug screening using the human tissue xenograft

After a potential therapeutic agent shows some activity in cultured tumor cell growth assays, its activity and toxicity are explored through *in vivo* xenograft models. Fragments of human tumors or cultured human tumor cells are implanted (often subcutaneously) into immunodeficient rodents. Once the tumors grow to a predetermined size, the potential anti-cancer agent is administered and the tumor response, generally assessed by tracking the tumor size, is measured over time. Drug doses and administration schedules are adjusted to optimize efficacy and to lower toxicity over several experimental cycles. This system generates valuable data and quickly returns a prediction on an agent's activity, often in several months. Unfortunately, promising anti-cancer compounds discovered through this route often fail in human clinical trials, commonly due to low efficacy (Kerbel et al., 2003; Sharpless & DePinho, 2006). The low predictive value of these xenograft models exemplifies the need for better *in vivo* mouse models for preclinical drug testing.

3. Birth of the transgenic "Oncomouse"

Transgenic mouse technology has evolved from the early 1980s (reviewed in Palmiter & Brinster, 1986) such that researchers can now conditionally and reversibly alter single gene expression. Thousands of publications have since supported the hypothesis that oncogene expression or tumor suppressor gene ablation in normal mammalian cells is sufficient to drive tumor development. The first report of a heritable tumor-prone transgenic mouse came in June 1984 (Brinster et al., 1984). These mice used the SV40 enhancer region to help drive expression of a construct consisting of the mouse metallothionein-1 gene promoter fused to the thymidine kinase gene from the herpes simplex virus (HSV). They included the whole SV40 upstream region, consisting of enhancer, promoter, and two T-antigen genes transcribed in the opposite direction. It was thought the T-antigen genes would be inactive in mice. Unexpectedly, they observed that the transgenic mice consistently developed brain tumors, as well as sporadic tumors in other tissues. Follow-up experiments showed that using only the SV40 enhancer/promoter region and the large T-antigen gene was sufficient to drive tumorigenesis (Palmiter et al., 1985). Subsequent reports have shown that expressing the large T-antigen in a specific cell type can promote tumor development. For example, Ornitz et al., (1985) demonstrated expression of the large T-antigen in acinar cells generated exocrine pancreatic tumors, whereas Hanahan (1985) used the insulin promoter driving the large T-antigen specifically in pancreatic beta-cells to produce endocrine pancreatic tumors.

Following the unexpected oncogenic ability of SV40, researchers tried to rationally design a tumor-generating transgenic mouse ("oncomouse"). In an effort to create a mouse model of a chromosomal translocation seen in some human B-cell lymphomas, Adams et al., (1985)

generated a transgene consisting of an immunoglobulin enhancer (Eμ) driving expression of the *Myc* gene. These mice heritably develop pre-B cell and mature B-cell lymphomas. Further studies by Strasser et al., (1990) showed that *Myc* required increased expression of the anti-apoptotic factor *Bcl-2* to drive tumorigenesis. Suppression of apoptosis is now understood to be a trademark of many cancer cells.

3.1 MMTV induced breast cancer

Using reciprocal matings between high tumor and low tumor mouse strains, Bittner (1936) reported tumor incidence in F1 females was dependent on the strain of the mother. Virologists demonstrated a virus (dubbed **M**urine **M**ammary **T**umor **V**irus, MMTV) was responsible for inducing tumors in mammary tissue and was passed from mother to offspring through her milk. Subsequent studies showed some mouse strains also had MMTV virus in their eggs and sperm (reviewed in Heston & Parks, 1977).

The utility of MMTV was expanded when it was shown that a short regulatory region (called long terminal repeat, LTR) was sufficient to confer hormone responsive and cell-specific expression *in vitro* (Huang et al., 1981). Stewart (1984) used the MMTV LTR to drive *Myc* expression in his transgenic mice that developed breast adenocarcinomas in mammary epithelial tissue. Since then the MMTV LTR has been fused with a variety of purported oncogenes to develop tumors in murine mammary tissue that are similar in morphology and gene expression profile to certain types of human breast cancers (reviewed in Robles & Varticovski, 2008). For example, the MMTV-driven **P**ol**y**oma **M**iddle-**T** antigen (*PyMT*) model develops tumors similar to a human breast cancer with luminal type morphology approximately 2-3 months after birth (Guy et al. 1992). A model expressing MMTV-driven *Wnt1* (wingless-type MMTV integration site family, member 1) generates mouse mammary tumors with characteristics similar to those of human basal type breast cancers (Huang et al., 2005). Several members of the *Wnt* gene family (encoding secretory glycoproteins that normally stimulate cell proliferation and differentiation) are expressed in the mouse mammary tissue during various stages of development. *Wnt-1* is not normally expressed in the mammary tissue; however, when driven ectopically by MMTV, it develops oncogenic properties. Like most of the other "first generation" transgenic oncomice, many of these models have a low tumor penetrance and widely variable latency period, making them difficult to use directly in large scale preclinical drug screenings. These limitations are partially overcome by resecting and transplanting transgenically induced tumors into many syngeneic recipient animals, generating a large cohort of tumor-bearing animals for drug-screening purposes (Maglione et al., 2004; Varticovski et al., 2007).

3.2 Activated kras

The KRAS2 gene encodes a G-protein that is a mammalian cellular homolog of a transforming gene isolated from the **K**irsten **RA**t **S**arcoma virus. This membrane-associated intracellular signal transducer plays a vital role in normal tissue signaling, proliferation, and differentiation (reviewed in Kranenburg, 2005). Several oncogenic point mutations interfere with the intrinsic GTPase activity of Kras, causing accumulation in a constitutively active GTP-bound state (Zenker et al., 2007). Expressing an activated *Kras* mutant transgene in acinar cells induces neoplasia in the fetal pancreas with large tumors developing only days after pancreatic differentiation (Quaife et al., 1987). Indeed, activating point mutations in the *Kras* gene have subsequently been shown to occur in 75 to 95% of spontaneous human pancreatic cancers (Almoguero et al., 1988) as well as > 90% of spontaneous and chemically induced mouse lung tumors (Malkinson 1998). Activated Kras expression in the mouse lung generates multiple tumors at an early age, so much so that the mice succumb quickly due to respiratory failure (Johnson et al., 2001). The varied penetrance and multi-focal primary tumor formation in addition to the short life span limits the use of this model in further studies of tumor development.

3.3 Knockout oncomice

The examples described thus far rely on the over expression of a nucleic acid sequence with purported oncogenic properties or mutations to drive tumorigenesis in mice. During the late 1980's the use of homologous recombination in mouse embryonic stem cells enabled researchers to inactivate ("knockout") single genes. This technology created a new wave of transgenic oncomice beginning with the heterozygous null retinoblastoma (Rb) mouse (Jacks et al., 1992). Rb inhibits the cell cycle by repressing expression of genes required for S phase progression (reviewed in Hanahan & Weiberg 2000). Mice lacking one Rb allele develop pituitary adenomas, whereas RB null offspring fail to develop beyond embryonic day 14 or 15, possibly due to excessive neuronal cell death.

The importance of tumor suppressor expression became evident from this and other knockout mouse models. Various cellular stresses prompt p53 to modulate expression of its target genes, many of which regulate cell cycle arrest, apoptosis, DNA repair, or cellular metabolism. Decreased or null expression of p53 has been observed in numerous human cancers (reviewed in Harris & Hollstein 1993). Mice lacking one or both p53 alleles are born normal but are predisposed to developing spontaneous lymphomas and sarcomas later in life (Donehower et al., 1992). Lacking a major tumor suppressor pathway, these p53 null mice became a useful background with which to elucidate the oncogenic potential of other genes. The Rb/p53 double knockout mice develop highly aggressive tumors in the cerebellum visible as early as 7 weeks of age (Marino et al., 2000). Mammary and skin tumors develop frequently in female mice carrying conditional null Brca2 and p53 alleles (Jonkers et al., 2001), suggesting synergistic inactivation of Brca2 and p53 can mediate mammary tumorigenesis.

Since these early transgenic and knockout mouse models have genetic alterations which are expressed in the germline and most, if not all, somatic cells, the models are more representative of human cancer predisposition syndromes. This is not the case for most human cancers, which develop spontaneously in a small number of cells in the adult. Many genes have distinct functions and expression patterns during embryonic development that are still poorly understood and different from those in the adult. In addition, these early transgenic models are notorious for their variable penetrance and tumor latency, making it nearly impossible to accumulate the number of animals with synchronous tumor development needed for large studies. While large scale production of transgenic mice is now possible with IVF and other high production methods (JAX® Speed Expansion Service; Charles River Laboratories Rapid Expansion Services), it does not obviate the issue of variable penetrance and tumor latency; it simply provides a large number of animals that can be held simultaneously to observe for tumor development. Early GEM models generated multiple primary lesions which far exceeded that observed in humans, limiting their predictive value and usefulness for preclinical studies. To better model most human cancers, genomic alterations should only occur in a small number of cells in the adult mouse tissue corresponding to the microenvironment in which the human cancer develops.

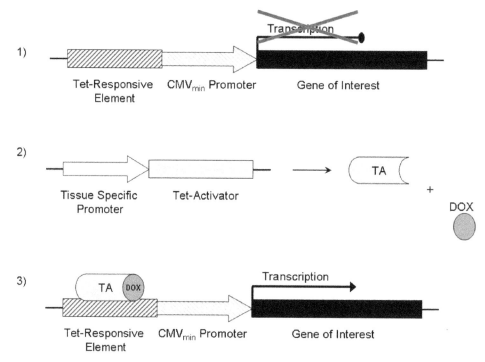

Fig. 2. Schematic Representation of the Tet-ON system; 1) Without the Tet-Activator (TA), the transgene consisting of the Gene-of-Interest (GOI) fused to the Tet-Responsive Element (TRE) will not be expressed. 2) Doxycycline can bind to the Tet-Activator protein, altering its protein structure such that TA can now bind to a TRE. 3) If both the Tet-Activator and the TRE-GOI transgenes are present in the same cell, upon doxycycline administration and TA activation, the GOI will be transcriptionally active.

4. Conditional and inducible oncogene expression

The ability to alter gene expression in a normal adult mouse overcomes many confounding factors gene manipulation might have in embryonic development and may better recapitulate human disease. A widely used inducible system is the Cre-Lox model (reviewed in Le & Sauer, 2001; Brault et al., 2007), where a segment of DNA is flanked by 34 base-pair (bp) LoxP sites (then referred to as floxed DNA). Co-expression of the Cre-recombinase (by crossbreeding with a tissue-specific Cre mouse (Nagy & Mar, 2001), or infecting with a virus carrying Cre) causes the region between the LoxP sequences to be spliced out (including all or part of the gene of interest) of the genome of that individual cell. Researchers have used this method to permanently silence genes in mice. There are two main limitations to the Cre-LoxP technology. The first obstacle is resolving how to administer Cre such that expression occurs only in the cells of interest. Crossing floxed mice with mice constitutively expressing Cre in a specific tissue often results in their offspring containing the deletion from the embryonic stage. It is difficult to administer Cre in the adult animal in a tissue-specific manner. The second limitation is the Cre-recombination event is irreversible and heritable.

To overcome some of these limitations, researchers have developed the Tet-ON/OFF system (reviewed in Sprengel & Hasan, 2007). It requires co-expression of two transgenes in a given cell, usually accomplished by cross-breeding. Driven by a user defined promoter, the first transgene generates the inactive Tetracycline Activator (TA). Doxycycline (a more potent isoform of the antibiotic tetracycline) can bind to and activate TA, which can bind the Tetracycline Response Element (TRE) on the second transgene and drive expression of its gene of interest (see Figure 2). Researchers use this system to initiate gene expression in adult animals through doxycycline administration in their chow. Since the oncogene expression is tied directly to the presence of doxycycline in their diet, the oncogene can be activated or silenced simply by adjusting an animal's diet. The main limitation to this procedure is the upfront time and labor needed to create mice that express the Tet-operator transgene and separate models expressing the tissue-specific Tet-activator transgene, then crossbreeding them to generate bi-transgenic offspring.

Both of these inducible expression systems can be used in reverse as well if the transgene constructs are designed accordingly. The Cre-recombinase can excise a multiple STOP cassette (Lox-STOP-Lox, LSL) integrated upstream of a transcription start site, enabling transcription of a previously silenced gene (see Figure 3). The Tet-ON/OFF system allows gene expression to be repeatedly induced or silenced in multiple cycles simply by providing or removing doxycycline from the animal's diet. However, the system was shown to be leaky in some early studies, resulting in incomplete expression inhibition or a low level of unregulated basal transcription. Adjunct technologies are continually being developed to obtain tighter gene expression control (reviewed in Freundlieb et al., 1999; Bockamp et al., 2007) which make these systems more robust, accurate, and thus more reliable as preclinical models. The following examples highlight the utility of inducible GEM tumor models.

4.1 Conditional cre-lox kras G12D system

Taking advantage of the Lox-Stop-Lox conditional transgene expression system, Jackson et al., (2001) created a transgenic mouse model which replaces one wild type *Kras* allele with a transcriptionally silent oncogenic Kras-G12D allele. Intranasally delivered adenovirus containing the Cre-recombinase (adeno-Cre) splices out the LSL and enables expression of the activated Kras-G12D transgene in the lung. Small lesions can be seen 2 weeks post induction; by 12 weeks post induction, adenomas are observed, some with cytogenic characteristics of malignancy. By 16 weeks post induction, large adenomas and adenocarcinomas are present in many animals. Virus titrations in a number of animals demonstrate that the number of virus particle equivalents used for induction is directly related to the number of tumors that develop.

Around the same time, Fisher et al., (2001) created an activated Kras Tet-ON/OFF inducible model. Doxycycline (DOX) administration induces expression of the murine oncogenic Kras G12D allele in alveolar type II pneumocytes. Hyperplasia is observed after just seven days of DOX administration; at eight weeks post induction, adenomas and adenocarcinomas are observed in the lungs. Removal of DOX from their diet causes a rapid decrease in activated Kras expression (within seven days) and apoptotic regression of the tumors. One month after DOX withdrawal, lesions and tumors were no longer present in the lungs, implying expression of the mutant Kras gene product was required to maintain the viability of tumor cells. The requirement of continued oncogene expression (or constant inhibition of tumor suppressor) to maintain the induced tumors has given rise to the theory of "oncogene addiction" (reviewed in Weinstein, 2002).

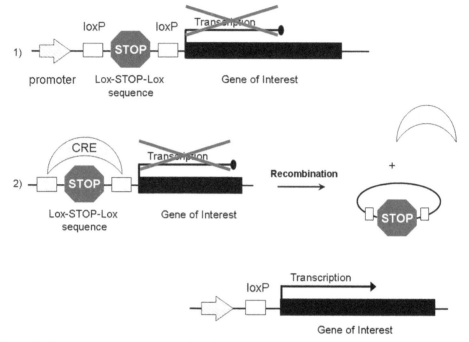

Fig. 3. CRE Recombination Mediates Lox-Stop-Lox Gene Activation. One popular method of inducing gene expression in adult mice is to use CRE recombination. 1) The transgenic mouse initially has the Lox-STOP-Lox sequence inserted upstream of the transcription start site for the gene of interest (GOI). This prevents GOI expression until acted upon by CRE. CRE recombinase is introduced to the appropriate cell population either by crossing with a second transgenic mouse expressing CRE recombinase using a tissue specific promoter, or by administering a virus expressing CRE recombinase in a tissue specific manner. 2) CRE recombinase splices out the STOP sequence between the two loxP sites from the transgenic DNA sequence, allowing GOI expression.

Sos et al., (2009) recently used computational genomic analysis to identify molecular and genetic predictors of therapeutic response to clinically relevant compounds in various NSCLC cancer cell lines which are highly representative of primary tumors. One of their findings was that cells expressing activated Kras also had enhanced Hsp90 dependency. They used the LSL-KrasG12D model to verify this observation. Mice were initially imaged by MRI 12-20 weeks post adeno-Cre administration, then split into placebo and 17-(Dimethylaminoethylamino)-17-demethoxygeldanamycin (17-DMAG a well-known Hsp90 inhibitor) groups. Mice were imaged by MRI after 1 week of drug treatment; tumor volume was decreased by 50% in 17-DMAG treated mice while tumor volume increased slightly in placebo treated animals. Prior to this study, there were no molecular targeted treatments for activated oncogenic Kras-driven lung tumors. But by combining the power of computational genomics and GEM models, researchers were able to rationally identify a possible therapeutic modality and evaluate its efficacy *in vivo*.

4.2 Inducible oncogenic mutations in the EGF receptor

The epidermal growth factor receptor (EGFr) is a transmembrane cell surface receptor which is mutated or alternatively expressed in a significant proportion of human gliomas and adenocarcinomas (especially of the head and neck, breast, colon, lung, and pancreas). EGFr is the human homolog of neu, a rat gene first identified in ethyl nitrosourea induced tumors (reviewed in Maguire & Greene, 1989), and is a member of the erythroblastic leukemia viral oncogene/human epidermal growth factor receptor (ERBB/HER) receptor tyrosine kinase family. Two of the most commonly observed EGFr mutations seen in lung adenocarcinomas include an in-frame deletion in exon 19 (eliminating an L-R-E-A [leucine-arginine-glutamic acid-alanine) amino acid motif that is conserved in all known vertebrate EGFr sequences) and a point mutation which results in a leucine to arginine substitution at position 858. These and other less common mutations in the kinase domain of EGFr are associated with increased therapeutic sensitivity to tyrosine kinase inhibitors such as gefitinib and erlotinib. Several studies demonstrated significantly extended survival and time to progression (TTP) in non-small-cell lung cancer (NSCLC) patients treated with gefitinib as their first line therapeutic (Han et al., 2005; Sequist et al., 2008; Yang et al., 2008). Erlotinib administration in patients who have had prior chemotherapy has an even greater survival benefit and is currently recommended by the FDA for second line therapy in new NSCLC patients (Shepherd et al., 2005). Inducible transgenic mouse models help to clarify this observation and provide a system to test other therapeutics that operate through the EGF receptor.

Politi et al., (2006) generated several Tet-ON/OFF mouse systems which overexpress various mutant EGFr alleles upon DOX administration. Lung adenocarcinomas were observed after two months post transgene induction in the exon 19 deletion and L858R transgenic EGFr mouse models. Similar to the Tet On/OFF activated Kras system, after one month of DOX withdrawal the observed tumor load in the EGFr transgene inducible models regressed to near pre-induction histology. To test the anti-tumor efficacy of an already clinically approved therapeutic in this model, the tyrosine kinase inhibitor erlotinib was administered to groups of transgenic EGFr mice maintained on DOX. After less than a week of erlotinib treatment, all of the animals which received at least 12 mg/kg/d showed partial or complete responses by magnetic resonance imaging (MRI). Longer lengths of treatment correlated with greater tumor regression. Ji et al., (2006) generated similar inducible EGFr transgenic mice (exon 19 in-frame deletion or L858R), but also added a luciferase fusion gene to the construct. This allows for the monitoring of lung tumor growth and regression *in vivo* using a non-invasive luciferase imaging system. The ability to non-invasively image tumor load repeatedly *in vivo* enables the effects of anti-cancer drug administration to be followed long term as the authors demonstrated with cetuximab.

4.3 GEMs possessing multiple genetic alterations

Patients with lung adenocarcinomas containing one of the common EGFr oncogenic mutations (deletion in exon 19 of the kinase domain [Del.ex19] and leucine 858 to arginine[L858R]) are sensitive to the EGFr-tyrosine kinase inhibitor (TKI) therapies (gefitinib and erlotinib). However, the TKI treated tumors invariably relapse within a year by developing resistance to the TKI therapy (reviewed in Morita et al., 2009), most commonly through one of the following mechanisms: EGFr-T790M point mutation (Kobayashi et al., 2005; Pao et al., 2005), MET proto-oncogene amplification (Engelman et al., 2007), or hyperphosphorylation and activation of insulin-like growth factor-I receptor (Guix et al., 2008). The EGFr-T790M mutation (observed in 50% of relapsed EGFr-mutant tumors) is thought to increase the ATP-binding affinity by an order of magnitude (Yun et al., 2008), thereby reducing the therapeutic ability of TKIs to out-compete ATP for receptor binding. MET amplification is thought to induce gefitinib resistance primarily by driving ERBB3 (HER3)-dependent activation of the PI3K and Erk pathways, which regulate cell survival and mitogenesis, respectively (reviewed in Kim & Salgia, 2009).

To overcome the acquired resistance of first generation TKIs, researchers have recently developed TKIs that bind EGFr irreversibly and are currently in or have completed phase II clinical trials (reviewed in Riely, 2008). The pan-ERBB inhibitor HKI-272 covalently binds to a cysteine in the EGFr kinase domain and regressed tumors at nanomolar concentrations in EGFR-L858R transgenic mice (Ji et al., 2006). The ability to inhibit ERBB2 (HER2) has led HKI-272 to be investigated primarily in breast cancer clinical trials (clinicaltrials.gov, 2011). However, other cancers driven by ErbB mutations may also be treated by HKI-272. Similarly, the irreversibly binding EGFr and HER2 inhibitor BIBW2992 is being tested in over 20 clinical trials of patients with advanced NSCLC, breast cancer, prostate cancer, malignant gliomas, and other solid tumors (clinicaltrials.gov, 2011). In addition to ERBB inhibitors, researchers are investigating other druggable targets related to the EGFr/HER2/ERK/AKT pathways. Shimamura et al., (2008) used an EGFR-L858R-T790M double transgenic GEM model to test the efficacy of an Hsp90 inhibitor, CL-387,785. Hsp90 is a chaperone thought to aid in the proper folding of EGFr; CL-387,785 binds irreversibly to Hsp90 thereby interfering with its chaperone function.

Cancer-related lethality in humans is often caused by the invasion of metastatic tumors in tissues far from the primary tumor. Yet few single transgene GEM models reliably develop metastatic lesions. By crossbreeding the pancreas-specific Cre-mediated activated Kras GEM (which alone generates only pre-malignant neoplasia) and the Ink4a/ARF conditional knockout models (does not induce neoplasia), Aguirre et al., (2003) generated mice that rapidly develop invasive, metastatic ductal pancreatic tumors which are lethal by 11 weeks. This tumor development is similar to the highly lethal human form of pancreatic ductal adenocarcinoma. Although the rapid murine mortality prevents long term studies, it may nevertheless be a useful model of a deadly human malignant cancer in short-term or cancer-prevention studies.

Similarly, Ji et al., (2007) crossed a lung-specific activated-Kras GEM with the following tumor suppressor knockout GEMs: Ink4a, p53, or the serine/threonine kinase 11 (Lkb1) knockout. Among the dual-knockout mice analyzed, the activated Kras x Lkb1 knockout had the most profound phenotype. These mice display a significantly increased lung tumor burden, rapid tumor onset, and <50% shorter survival when compared to the other double crosses or single knockout models examined. Regional lymph-node metastases were observed in 61% of the activated Kras x Lkb1 knockout mice, significantly more than the other models. The results from the previous few examples suggest an activating Kras mutation is responsible for initial neoplasia development, but a second mutated gene modulates the aggressiveness and metastatic behavior of the cancer. Accumulation of somatic mutations over time has long been a theory to explain the modulation and late onset of cancer in humans.

Winslow et al., (2011) expanded on this idea by administering a lentivirus expressing Cre recombinase to a double floxed GEM model. Upon CRE recombination, activated Kras would be expressed and p53 (flox/flox) would be silenced in certain cells of the adult lung. Because the lentivirus integrates randomly into the host cell's genome, the authors were able to use linkage-mediated PCR (LM-PCR) to generate a unique "fingerprint" for each primary tumor and monitor that "fingerprint" in any subsequent metastases. Although virus was delivered at a set time point and many primary foci seemed to successfully undergo the oncogenic double recombination event, only a few primary foci were responsible for generating macroscopic metastases outside the lung, suggesting other genetic or micro-environmental factors control a tumor's metastatic potential. This is an excellent example of using an inducible, double GEM to model genetic alterations seen in many human lung cancers and explore the genetics of malignant and non-malignant tumors.

Tp53 is not the only tumor suppressor being actively investigated using GEM models. The tumor suppressor phosphatase and tensin homologue (PTEN) is a lipid phosphatase which negatively regulates the PI3/AKT pathway, which is often upregulated in human malignancies. Sixty percent of primary human prostate cancers show a decrease/loss of PTEN expression; this gene also is deleteriously mutated in 70% of gliomas and in some forms of breast carcinomas and melanomas (Gray et al., 1998). To investigate the role of PTEN in prostate cancer, Trotman et al., (2003) created several PTEN GEM models, each with a different level of PTEN expression. Only the homozygous PTEN knockout show a significant phenotype (invasive prostate cancer develops after six months in all mice). However, none of the models generate metastases and the mice do not have decreased survival compared to wild type controls. A prostate-specific PTEN conditional knockout was created which also generated invasive prostate cancer; but in this case metastatic prostate tumors developed and were found in the lymph and lung (Wang et al., 2003). Concomitant inactivation of one or both Cdkn1b (encodes the tumor suppressor p27) alleles in a heterozygous PTEN knockout mouse accelerates spontaneous neoplasia formation which develop into prostate carcinoma at complete penetrance within three months from birth (Di Cristofano et al., 2001). When a conditional PTEN knockout mouse is crossed with a p53 knockout mouse the resulting offspring is a conditional double knockout GEM that develops aggressive, lethal prostate cancer with complete penetrance in seven months (Chen et al., 2005). The cancers observed in this new generation of GEM models recapitulate the progression and histopathologic features of some forms of prostate cancer observed in humans. These studies highlight the role of PTEN in tumorigenesis and the need for additional cooperative tumor suppressor inactivation to generate malignancies and lethal cancers.

The potential for drug discovery and validation using conditional GEM models is demonstrated with the Brca1/p53 mouse model. The majority of human BRCA1-associated tumors harbor mutations in both p53 and BRCA1. Poole et al., (2006) created such a Cre-LoxP conditional GEM model by inactivating both p53 and Brca1 specifically in the mouse mammary gland. The authors found that progesterone receptors are overexpressed in mutant mammary epithelial cells and presented a possible avenue of treatment. Administration of a progesterone agonist (mifepristone, RU 486) prevented mammary tumorigenesis in Brca1/p53-deficient mice. As the potential to genotype a patient's tumor to determine their status for EGFr, MET, p53, IGF, and other important neoplasia-associated targets becomes practical, it will be possible to better choose the optimal combination therapy to impact the relevant oncogenic pathways.

5. The predictive potential of GEMs

The potential predictive power of transgenic mice can be illustrated in the example of thiazolidinediones (TZDs). As an agonist of peroxisome proliferator-activated receptor-gamma (PPARγ), the TZD troglitazone had been an FDA-approved therapy for type-2 diabetes. TZD anti-tumor activity in cultured and xenografted human colon cancer cells prompted excitement in the scientific community that initiated its use in Phase II clinical trials in patients with colon cancer (Sarraf et al., 1998). However, in a study published a few pages after the xenograft study, troglitazone showed no anti-tumor activity in Min+/- mice; in fact, polyp formation increased with troglitazone administration in this model (Saez et al., 1998). This heterozygous knockout mouse model lacks one functional copy of the APC tumor suppresser gene, thus predisposing them to colon cancer. In the Phase II clinical trial patients treated with troglitazone actually showed disease progression within months of therapy initiation, correlating with the results predicted from the transgenic mouse model (Kulke et al., 2002).

5.1 Cautionary tale

Although many regard mice as "little fuzzy humans" in the analysis of preclinical data, there are vast and often unknown differences in drug metabolism, gene expression, and disease progression between the murine model and humans. One example of transgenic mouse models failing to accurately predict human clinical outcome is the Farnesyltransferase (FTase) story. FTase catalyzes the post-translational farnesylation of proteins containing a C-terminal CAAX motif, where C is the cysteine residue to be farnesylated, A represents an aliphatic amino acid, and X is any amino acid. When X is leucine, the protein is a preferred substrate for a similar enzyme named geranylgeranyltransferase I (GGTase).

Mendola & Backer, (1990) showed farnesylation of Ras proteins is critical for their transformation into potent oncogenes. This discovery ignited the hypothesis that interfering with prenylation using inhibitors of FTase (FTIs) or GGTase (GGTIs) could lead to tumor growth inhibition and a viable anti-cancer therapy. Although some data suggest an FTI and a GGTI need to be utilized simultaneously to achieve complete inhibition of Kras prenylation (Rowell et al., 1997), FTIs alone had been shown to inhibit growth of human tumor xenografts in nude mice (Sun et al., 1998). FTI monotherapy also demonstrates beneficial effects in transgenic mouse models: tumor regression in H-Ras mice (Kohl et al., 1995), tumor stasis in N-Ras mice (Mangues et al., 1998), and tumor growth inhibition in Ki-RasB mice (Omer et al., 2000). These results and others spurred excitement for FTI monotherapy in clinical trials. With the exception of a few trials in breast cancer and leukemia patients, FTIs used as single agents have not shown good efficacy against solid tumors (reviewed in Zhu et al., 2003). Thus, none of the various mouse models evaluated were able to predict drug efficacy in humans. However, many clinical trials are currently underway combining FTIs with other drugs including "classical" anticancer therapies (chemotherapy or radiotherapy) and molecular targeted therapeutics.

5.2 Targeted molecular therapeutics

For decades, cancer therapy has been one or a combination of the following three treatments: surgery, radiotherapy, and cytotoxic chemotherapy. However, all have their limitations and substantial side effects. Ideally, anti-cancer treatments would "target" cancer cells and minimize adverse effects to non-cancerous cells. Tumors often contain gene expression profiles and mutations that make them more or less sensitive to some targeted therapies than others. Identifying the tumor's gene expression profile and correlating it to the most successful therapies for that specific profile will keep therapeutic adverse side effects to a minimum and yield the best prognosis for the patient.

The two main types of targeted molecular therapies are monoclonal antibodies, which target the receptor's extracellular domain, and small molecule inhibitors, which target the intracellular signaling and kinase domains. Table 1 outlines some of the FDA-approved targeted therapeutics, their molecular targets, and the forms of cancer in which they have been proven to have a clinical benefit. Monoclonal antibodies (mabs) are generally administered no more than once weekly by intravenous injection, whereas small molecules (nibs) can generally be taken orally each day. Currently available targeted therapies may be administered as single agents, but many show greater benefits in combination with other agents or in addition to traditional therapies in those patient populations with tumors of susceptible genetic profiles. Tumors can be generated in genetically engineered mice which have these susceptible mutations and expression profiles, providing researchers with valuable preclinical drug screening opportunities.

Herceptin (HER2) is a transmembrane receptor that is over-expressed in 20-25% of breast cancers and is associated with aggressive tumor behavior and poor prognosis (reviewed in Nanda, 2007). Two early studies have shown the anti-HER2 monoclonal antibody trastuzumab plus chemotherapy significantly improves overall survival in HER2+ patients with metastatic breast cancer (Slamon et al., 2005). Antibody binding is thought to inhibit HER2 signaling, which disrupts DNA repair mechanisms and induces cytotoxicity. Resistance to trastuzumab commonly occurs and can render this treatment useless in subsequent relapses. A recent advance has been to conjugate the antibody with a toxin/drug, thereby creating a "guided missile" that targets a specific epitope over-expressed on cancer cells and delivers the toxic agent to those specific cells. Researchers at Genetech harvested mammary tumors from MMTV-HER2 transgenic mice, implanted them orthotopically into a large cohort of nude mice, staged the mice when mean tumor volumes were ~100-200 mm^3, and administered their trastuzumab-DM1 (T-DM1) conjugate at various time points and doses (Jumbe et al., 2010). DM1, also known as maytansine and derived from members of several tropical plant families, is a potent cytotoxin that irreversibly inhibits tubulin polymerization and arrests cells in M or G2 phase (Remillard et al., 1975; Rao et al., 1979). Because the toxin is specifically targeted to tumor cells, the authors saw no adverse events in the mice, with ~50% of the tumors showing complete regression at doses of 15 mg/kg given once every three weeks. PD/PK measures were obtained from the mice and this immunoconjugate therapy is now being evaluated in several clinical trials in patients with metastatic breast cancer.

Several therapeutics have been developed that target the EGFr receptor to treat non-small cell lung cancer and colorectal cancer, including cetuximab, panitumumab, erlotinib, and gefitinib. Tumors expressing EGFr with a deletion in exon 19 or sensitizing point mutation (L858R) in the ATP-binding pocket respond significantly better to gefitinib than patients with wild type EGFr (Lynch et al., 2008). Invariably, even the tumors with increased drug sensitivity relapse when resistance to gefitinib develops. Additional therapeutics need to be generated to overcome the inevitable drug resistance.

Targeted Therapy	Molecular Target	Approved Use
cetuximab (Erbitux®)	EGFr	Colorectal Cancer
erlotinib (Tarceva®)	EGFr	Non-Small Cell Lung Cancer Metastatic Pancreatic Cancer
gefitinib (Iressa®)	EGFr	Non-Small Cell Lung Cancer
panitumumab (Vectibix®)	EGFr	Colorectal Cancer
trastuzumab (Herceptin®)	HER2	Early and Metastatic Breast Cancer
lapatinib (Tykerb®)	HER2 and EGFr	Breast Cancer
bevacizumab (Avastin®)	VEGF	Metastatic Colorectal Cancer Metastatic Melanoma Non-Small Cell Lung Cancer
sunitinib (Sutent®)	VEGFr and PDGFr	Metastatic Renal Cell Carcinoma
sorafenib (Nexavar®)	Multi-Targeted Kinase Inhibitor	Metastatic Renal Cell Carcinoma
toceranib (Palladia®)	Multi-Targeted Kinase Inhibitor	Canine Specific Mastocytoma
pazopanib (Votrient®)	VEGFr, PDGFr, and cKIT	Advanced Renal Cell Carcinoma
imatinib (Gleevec®)	cKIT, ABL, and PDGFr2	Chronic Myeloid Leukemia and GIST
dasatinib (Sprycel®)	BCR/ABL and Src Family	Chronic Myeloid Leukemia with resistance to prior therapy
alemtuzumab (Campath®, MabCampath® or Campath-1H®)	CD52 on Mature Lymphocytes	Chronic Lymphocytic Leukemia (CLL) and Cutaneous T-cell Lymphoma (CTCL)
ofatumumab (Arzerra®)	CD20 on B-cells	Chronic Lymphocytic Leukemia (CLL)
rituximab (MabThera® and Rituxan®)	CD20 on B-cells	B-cell Non-Hodgkin's Lymphoma
nilotinib (Tasigna®)	BCR/ABL kinase inhibitor	Philadelphia chromosome positive chronic myeloid leukemia (CML)
vandetanib (Zactima®)	VEGFr, EGFr, RET	Metastatic Medullary Thyroid Cancer

EGFr: Epidermal growth factor receptor;erythroblastic leukemia viral (v-erb-b) oncogene homolog 1
VEGFr: Vascular endothelial growth factor receptor
PDGFr2: Platelet-derived growth factor receptor-alpha
BCR/ABL: c-abl oncogene 1, receptor tyrosine kinase
cKIT: v-kit Hardy-Zuckerman 4 feline sarcoma viral oncogene homolog
Her2: Herceptin receptor; v-erb-b2 erythroblastic leukemia viral oncogene homolog 2
RET: "Rearranged during transfection" proto oncogene

Table 1. An overview of the currently FDA approved targeted therapy compounds.

Since vascularization is required for growth and health of a tumor, the angiogenesis associated factor VEGF became a desired target for therapy. Bevacizumab is an anti-VEGF antibody which has been shown to bind and inhibit VEGF, slowing angiogenesis and aiding in solid tumor starvation and elimination (Brekken et al., 2000). When used as single agents in unsorted cancer patients, anti-angiogenic therapeutics do not show significant activity. However, when used in combination with other therapies (especially cytotoxic chemotherapy), subgroups of patients show promise (reviewed in Cabebe, 2007). Bevacizumab, in addition to paclitaxel and a platinum cytotoxic agent, is now part of a first line therapy for newly diagnosed non-small cell lung cancer. Hundreds of Phase II and Phase III trials using bevacizumab in combination with other therapies in many other cancers are currently ongoing (clinicaltrials.gov, 2011).

5.3 GEM oncomice in cancer prevention
GEM models are beginning to realize their potential as preclinical models of cancer prevention (briefly reviewed in Abate-Shen et al., 2008). In a recent example, Ohashi et al., (2009) used the EGFR-L858R-FLAG transgenic mouse to test the cancer preventative potential of gefitinib administration. Twenty-five 3-week old transgenic mice were administered gefitinib, with 5, 5, and 15 mice euthanized at weeks 8, 13, and 18, respectively. At termination the lungs tumors were counted and measured macroscopically and histologically. Those receiving gefitinib failed to develop adenocarcinomas, whereas the groups given vehicle control developed hyperplastic regions at 5 weeks and large adenocarcinomas by 15 weeks. One week after cessation of the 15-week gefitinib administration period, the transgenic mice showed signs of hyperplastic cell expansion in the lung (by PCNA staining), suggesting gefitinib was the lone factor preventing EGFr-L858R tumor development in these mice. Longer term studies are needed to see if the EGFr-L858R transgenic mice eventually develop gefitinib resistance, as is seen in human NCSLC patients with EGFr-L858R driven lung tumors. Similar studies with erlotinib, other tyrosine kinase inhibitors, and novel anti-cancer agents should be performed on this and other informative GEM models to further investigate the tumor-preventative aspects of these agents.

5.4 Cancer vaccine
It is conceivable that patients with a high risk (family history, environmental exposure, or heritable mutations) associated with a specific cancer subtype might benefit from being immunized at a young age. Vaccine development depends on the identification of antigens specific for a given cancer subtype or tumor-inducing biological agent. The heterogeneity and unstable genome in most cancers suggests resistant mutant cells might accumulate quickly and overcome the immunotherapy. However, vaccines against oncogenic strains of viruses have proven to be very beneficial and often lean on the preclinical use of GEM models to show the oncogenic potential of viral genes.
In 1993, two studies using transgenic mice emerged clearly showing the oncogenic potential of the human papillomavirus (HPV) early genes E6 and E7 (Lambert et al., 1993; Arbeit et al., 1993). HPV DNA has also been found in and hypothesized by some to induce a subset of tongue and other oropharyngeal carcinomas (reviewed in Syrjänen, 2005). Transgenic mice expressing HPV early genes have been used to demonstrate the oncogenic potential of HPV in certain skin cancers [HPV 8 (Schaper et al., 2005) and HPV 20 (Michel et al., 2006)]. Spurred by these and many studies elucidating the relationship between HPV and cervical

cancer, the FDA approved the HPV vaccine Gardasil (Merck) for preventing the most common forms of human papillomavirus (HPV)-induced cervical cancer (reviewed in McLemore, 2006). Feng et al., (2008) recently discovered a novel polyomavirus (similar to SV40) that integrated itself into the genome of 80% of the Merkel cell carcinomas they examined. Though a rare cancer, this is another example of a virus-associated cancer which could be a target for cancer-preventing vaccines and could be tested preclinically in GEM models.

5.5 Legal obstacles of preclinical testing in GEM models

In 1988 Harvard University filed the first of three exceptionally broad U.S. patents regarding the development and use of transgenic animals. Dupont (a sponsor of one of the Harvard investigators developing transgenic mice) became the exclusive licensee of transgenic patents and merely sublicensed the patent rights (imposing large fees and restrictions) to industry and academia. This arrangement severely constrained use of transgenic mice beyond basic discovery applications (reviewed in Sharpless & Depinho, 2006). Fortunately for the greater scientific community, the first of these patents expired in 2005 and the second expired in February 2009; the third patent covering testing methods using transgenic oncomice is still in force through 2016. Hundreds of oncomice have been developed (primarily in academia), but have yet to be thoroughly studied and used on a large scale to test the growing number of possible anti-cancer therapies. Once the final restriction is lifted, researchers in industry, academia, and government alike will undoubtedly expand their use of transgenic models for preclinical drug studies.

6. Conclusion: Role GEMs can play in preclinical studies

To process the thousands of novel natural product and synthetic purported anti-cancer compounds that arise each year, preclinical drug screens must be as quick and comprehensive as resources allow. This can best be accomplished by *in vitro* screens using cultured cell lines that have oncogenic gene expression profiles similar to those seen in human patients. Compounds which show activity can then be moved to xenograft studies, which test toxicity and tumor regression potential. Although we have reviewed the power of GEM models in verifying drug efficacy and pathway mechanism analysis, GEM models as they exist today have fundamental flaws that preclude their use as high-throughput drug-screening tools.

GEMs require several months to develop tumors, and the penetrance is often far less than 100%. Tumors arise and grow at different rates in each individual mouse in a given study. Except for melanoma, breast cancer, and some prostate cancer models where palpable tumors develop, identifying which animals have developed tumors at any given moment becomes a nearly insurmountable task. Many published studies use MRI images to follow tumor progression. Considering imaging the thorax of one mouse in an MRI can take up to one hour, this method is incompatible with large, high throughput studies. Small animal in vivo imaging (SAIVI) using fluorescent or bioluminescent tagged agents targeting tumors is a promising alternative, but the technology is still in its infancy, lacks appropriate inducible GEM models for most forms of cancer, and often requires purchase of expensive, photosensitive probes and detection systems. Computed Tomography (CT) Imaging with clinical-size instruments cannot be used because the dose of radiation used during imaging may have therapeutic effects on the tumors, especially when GEM models will require multiple imaging sessions over their lifetime to first identify a tumor and then to monitor therapeutic drug effects. However as smaller, less powerful, rodent-specific CT imagers become available to researchers, this may prove to be a useful method to measure tumor size in deep tissue. To best utilize current GEM models in preclinical drug trials, traditional tumor staging strategies must be revised so that each mouse is treated as a patient in a clinical trial. Therapeutic agents must not be administered en mass to all individuals in a treatment group at a given time point, but tailored to each mouse reflecting the date the tumor was recognized by whatever modality the researcher has developed. This can create a logistical nightmare, especially if large combination therapy treatment trials testing multiple vehicles, routes of administration, dosing schedules, and multiple dose concentrations are attempted. Day 0 should be marked at the time an animal's measured tumor size or total "tumor burden" (if the GEM generates multiple foci simultaneously) crosses a pre-determined threshold quantity.

Therefore, we cannot envision GEM models replacing *in vitro* and xenograft models for the high throughput efficacy screens of novel agents. However, we do believe GEM models can be of great value during three steps in the preclinical process (Figure 1). First, if GEM tumors are harvested and fragments successfully implanted subcutaneously (SC) or orthotopically into syngeneic, immune competent mice, enough animals can be amassed to perform traditional xenograft-like screens with genetically desirable murine tumors (allografts). Varticovski et al., (2007) provide an example of this approach, harvesting MMTV-PyMT breast tumors from a few mice and passing them as fragments or cell suspensions into numerous host animals for subsequent drug studies. DNA microarrays were used to verify only slight changes in gene expression after two serial passages from the original tumor. Second passage tumors exhibited similar sensitivity to paclitaxel and cyclophosphamide compared to the original tumor material.

Once an agent shows activity *in vitro* and in tumor transplants, GEM models can be used to explore the drug mechanism and further optimize *in vivo* dosing before an agent heads into the much more expensive and laborious clinical trials (Figure 1). These optimization studies need not be high throughput and may take a year or more to complete. Thus, fewer anti-cancer agents will successfully pass through these additional preclinical evaluations than do currently advance to clinical trial. Currently, only ~5% of novel anti-cancer agents entering clinical trials achieve FDA approval (Kola & Landis, 2004); most of the cost and attrition occurs during Phase II and Phase III clinical trials. Therefore any extra time GEM-based drug screening would add to the preclinical drug development pipeline should be financially worthwhile to the drug sponsors and ethically beneficial for the volunteers participating in clinical trials if more efficacious therapies are discovered.

GEM models may ultimately have a fourth role in preclinical drug testing if researchers can effectively "humanize" them for use in toxicology and pharmacology studies. The cytochrome P450 (CYP) family of enzymes are expressed primarily in the liver and are involved in the metabolism of a diverse range of therapeutic compounds, toxins, carcinogens, hormones, and xenobiotic agents we may encounter. The seven main CYP gene clusters found in humans are present and expanded in mice (57 putative human CYP genes versus 102 putative functional genes in mice) (Nelson et al., 2004). But studies have shown that many individual CYPs are differentially expressed or differentially active between the mouse and human (Bogaards et al., 2000). This explains why drug metabolism in the mouse does not always reflect and predict drug metabolism and toxicity in the human clinical trials. Several GEM models have been generated in which the endogenous mouse CYPs or other xenobiotic-related metabolism genes are deleted and replaced with their human orthologues, or simply over express the human orthologue in addition to the mouse CYP (reviewed in Cheung & Gonzalez, 2008). Expression of one or two human genes certainly is not enough to declare a potential GEM model as functionally "humanized" and ready for high throughput toxicity and pharmacology studies. But as transgenic technology evolves and these mice express numerous human orthologues, they may indeed be able to better predict human drug activity and toxicity, and be of vital importance in preclinical therapeutic drug development.

7. References

Abate-Shen C, Brown PH, Colburn NH, Gerner EW, Green JE, Lipkin M, Nelson WG, Threadgill D. (2008). The untapped potential of genetically engineered mouse models in chemoprevention research: opportunities and challenges. *Cancer Prev Res (Phila Pa)*. 1(3):161-6.

Adams JM, Harris AW, Pinkert CA, Corcoran LM, Alexander WS, Cory S, Palmiter RD, Brinster RL. (1985). The c-myc oncogene driven by immunoglobulin enhancers induces lymphoid malignancy in transgenic mice. *Nature*. 318(6046):533-8.

Aguirre AJ, Bardeesy N, Sinha M, Lopez L, Tuveson DA, Horner J, Redston MS, DePinho RA. (2003). Activated Kras and Ink4a/Arf deficiency cooperate to produce metastatic pancreatic ductal adenocarcinoma. *Genes Dev*. 17(24):3112-26.

Almoguera, C.; Shibata, D.; Forrester, K.; Martin, J.; Arnheim, N.; Perucho, M. (1988). Most human carcinomas of the exocrine pancreas contain mutant c-K-ras genes. *Cell*. 53: 549-554.

American Cancer Society (ACS). (2010). Cancer Facts & Figures 2010. Atlanta: American Cancer Society.

Arbeit JM, Münger K, Howley PM, Hanahan D. (1993). Neuroepithelial carcinomas in mice transgenic with human papillomavirus type 16 E6/E7 ORFs. *Am J Pathol*. 142(4):1187-97.

Bittner JJ. Some possible effects of nursing on the mammary gland tumor incidence in mice. *Science*. 1936; 84:162.

Bockamp E, Christel C, Hameyer D, Khobta A, Maringer M, Reis M, Heck R, Cabezas-Wallscheid N, Epe B, Oesch-Bartlomowicz B, Kaina B, Schmitt S, Eshkind L. (2007). Generation and characterization of tTS-H4: a novel transcriptional repressor that is compatible with the reverse tetracycline-controlled TET-ON system. *J Gene Med*. 9(4):308-18.

Bogaards JJ, Bertrand M, Jackson P, Oudshoorn MJ, Weaver RJ, van Bladeren PJ, Walther B. (2000). Determining the best animal model for human cytochrome P450 activities: a comparison of mouse, rat, rabbit, dog, micropig, monkey and man. *Xenobiotica*. 30(12):1131-52.

Brault V, Besson V, Magnol L, Duchon A, Hérault Y. (2007). Cre/loxP-mediated chromosome engineering of the mouse genome. *Handb Exp Pharmacol*. (178):29-48.

Brekken RA, Overholser JP, Stastny VA, Waltenberger J, Minna JD, Thorpe PE. (2000). Selective inhibition of vascular endothelial growth factor (VEGF) receptor 2

(KDR/Flk-1) activity by a monoclonal anti-VEGF antibody blocks tumor growth in mice. *Cancer Res.* 60(18):5117-24.

Brinster RL, Chen HY, Messing A, van Dyke T, Levine AJ, Palmiter RD. (1984). Transgenic mice harboring SV40 T-antigen genes develop characteristic brain tumors. *Cell.* 37(2):367-79.

Cabebe E and Wakelee H. (2007). Role of anti-angiogenesis agents in treating NSCLC: focus on bevacizumab and VEGFR tyrosine kinase inhibitors. *Curr Treat Options Oncol.* 8(1):15-27.

Charles River Laboratories Rapid Expansion Services. (2006). In: *Assisted Reproductive Technologies.* Charles River Laboratories. 1 July 2011. Available from: <http://www.criver.com/sitecollectiondocuments/rm_tg_d_sperm_ovarian_cryo preservation.pdf>

Chen Z, Trotman LC, Shaffer D, Lin HK, Dotan ZA, Niki M, Koutcher JA, Scher HI, Ludwig T, Gerald W, Cordon-Cardo C, Pandolfi PP. (2005). Crucial role of p53-dependent cellular senescence in suppression of Pten-deficient tumorigenesis. *Nature.* 436(7051):725-30.

Cheung C, Gonzalez FJ. (2008). Humanized mouse lines and their application for prediction of human drug metabolism and toxicological risk assessment. *J Pharmacol Exp Ther.* 327(2):288-99.

Clinicaltrials.gov. n.d. *U.S. National Institutes of Health.* 1 July 2011. Available from: <http://www.clinicaltrials.gov/ct2/home>

Decker S, Hollingshead M, Bonomi CA, Carter JP, Sausville EA. (2004). The hollow fibre model in cancer drug screening: the NCI experience. *Eur J Cancer.* 40(6):821-6.

Di Cristofano A, De Acetis M, Koff A, Cordon-Cardo C, Pandolfi PP. (2001). Pten and p27KIP1 cooperate in prostate cancer tumor suppression in the mouse. *Nat Genet.* 27(2):222-4.

Donehower LA, Harvey M, Slagle BL, McArthur MJ, Montgomery CA Jr, Butel JS, Bradley A. (1992). Mice deficient for p53 are developmentally normal but susceptible to spontaneous tumours. *Nature.* 356(6366):215-21.

eMICE. electronic Models Information, Communication, and Education. n.d. National Cancer Institute. 1 July 2011. Available from: <http://emice.nci.nih.gov/acquiring-models/Mice>

Engelman JA, Zejnullahu K, Mitsudomi T, Song Y, Hyland C, Park JO, Lindeman N, Gale CM, Zhao X, Christensen J, Kosaka T, Holmes AJ, Rogers AM, Cappuzzo F, Mok T, Lee C, Johnson BE, Cantley LC, Jänne PA. (2007). MET amplification leads to gefitinib resistance in lung cancer by activating ERBB3 signaling. *Science.* 316(5827):1039-43.

Feng H, Shuda M, Chang Y, Moore PS. (2008). Clonal integration of a polyomavirus in human Merkel cell carcinoma. Science. 319(5866):1096-100.

Fisher GH, Wellen SL, Klimstra D, Lenczowski JM, Tichelaar JW, Lizak MJ, Whitsett JA, Koretsky A, Varmus HE. (2001). Induction and apoptotic regression of lung adenocarcinomas by regulation of a K-Ras transgene in the presence and absence of tumor suppressor genes. *Genes Dev.* 15(24):3249-62.

Freundlieb S, Schirra-Müller C, Bujard H. (1999). A tetracycline controlled activation/repression system with increased potential for gene transfer into mammalian cells. *J Gene Med.* 1(1):4-12.

Gray IC, Stewart LM, Phillips SM, Hamilton JA, Gray NE, Watson GJ, Spurr NK, Snary D. (1998). Mutation and expression analysis of the putative prostate tumour-suppressor gene PTEN. *Br J Cancer.* 78(10):1296-300.

Guix M, Faber AC, Wang SE, Olivares MG, Song Y, Qu S, Rinehart C, Seidel B, Yee D, Arteaga CL, Engelman JA. (2008). Acquired resistance to EGFR tyrosine kinase inhibitors in cancer cells is mediated by loss of IGF-binding proteins. *J Clin Invest.* 118(7):2609-19.

Guy CT, Cardiff RD, Muller WJ. (1992). Induction of mammary tumors by expression of polyomavirus middle T oncogene: a transgenic mouse model for metastatic disease. *Mol Cell Biol.* 12(3):954-61.

Han SW, Kim TY, Hwang PG, Jeong S, Kim J, Choi IS, Oh DY, Kim JH, Kim DW, Chung DH, Im SA, Kim YT, Lee JS, Heo DS, Bang YJ, Kim NK. (2005). Predictive and prognostic impact of epidermal growth factor receptor mutation in non-small-cell lung cancer patients treated with gefitinib. *J Clin Oncol.* 23(11):2493-501.

Hanahan D. (1985). Heritable formation of pancreatic beta-cell tumours in transgenic mice expressing recombinant insulin/simian virus 40 oncogenes. *Nature.* 315(6015):115-22.

Hanahan D and Weinberg RA. (2000). The hallmarks of cancer. *Cell.* 100: 57-70.

Harris CC and Hollstein M. (1993). Clinical implications of the p53 tumor-suppressor gene. *New Eng. J. Med.* 329: 1318-1327.

Heston WE and Parks WP. (1977). Mammary tumors and mammary tumor virus expression in hybrid mice of strains C57BL and GR. *J. Exp. Med.* 146: 1206-1220.

Huang AL, Ostrowski MC, Berard D, Hager GL. (1981). Glucocorticoid regulation of the Ha-MuSV p21 gene conferred by sequences from mouse mammary tumor virus. *Cell.* 27(2 Pt 1):245-55.

Huang S, Li Y, Chen Y, Podsypanina K, Chamorro M, Olshen AB, Desai KV, Tann A, Petersen D, Green JE, Varmus HE. (2005). Changes in gene expression during the development of mammary tumors in MMTV-Wnt-1 transgenic mice. *Genome Biol.* 6(10):R84.

Jacks T, Fazeli A, Schmitt EM, Bronson RT, Goodell MA, Weinberg RA. (1992). Effects of an Rb mutation in the mouse. *Nature.* 359(6393):295-300.

Jackson EL, Willis N, Mercer K, Bronson RT, Crowley D, Montoya R, Jacks T, Tuveson DA. (2001). Analysis of lung tumor initiation and progression using conditional expression of oncogenic K-ras. *Genes Dev.* 15(24):3243-8.

JAX® Speed Expansion Service. n.d. *The Jackson Laboratory.* 1 July 2011. Available from: <http://jaxservices.jax.org/breeding/speed-expansion.html>

Ji H, Li D, Chen L, Shimamura T, Kobayashi S, McNamara K, Mahmood U, Mitchell A, Sun Y, Al-Hashem R, Chirieac LR, Padera R, Bronson RT, Kim W, Jänne PA, Shapiro GI, Tenen D, Johnson BE, Weissleder R, Sharpless NE, Wong KK. (2006). The impact of human EGFR kinase domain mutations on lung tumorigenesis and in vivo sensitivity to EGFR-targeted therapies. *Cancer Cell.* 9(6):485-95.

Ji H, Ramsey MR, Hayes DN, Fan C, McNamara K, Kozlowski P, Torrice C, Wu MC, Shimamura T, Perera SA, Liang MC, Cai D, Naumov GN, Bao L, Contreras CM, Li D, Chen L, Krishnamurthy J, Koivunen J, Chirieac LR, Padera RF, Bronson RT, Lindeman NI, Christiani DC, Lin X, Shapiro GI, Jänne PA, Johnson BE, Meyerson M, Kwiatkowski DJ, Castrillon DH, Bardeesy N, Sharpless NE, Wong KK. (2007). LKB1 modulates lung cancer differentiation and metastasis. *Nature.* 448(7155): 807-10.

Johnson L, Mercer K, Greenbaum D, Bronson RT, Crowley D, Tuveson DA, and Jacks T. (2001). Somatic activation of the K-ras oncogene causes early onset lung cancer in mice. *Nature.* 410: 1111–1116.

Jonkers J, Meuwissen R, van der Gulden H, Peterse H, van der Valk M, Berns A. (2001). Synergistic tumor suppressor activity of BRCA2 and p53 in a conditional mouse model for breast cancer. *Nature Genet.* 29: 418-425.

Jumbe NL, Xin Y, Leipold DD, Crocker L, Dugger D, Mai E, Sliwkowski MX, Fielder PJ, Tibbitts J. (2010). Modeling the efficacy of trastuzumab-DM1, an antibody drug conjugate, in mice. *J Pharmacokinet Pharmacodyn.* 37(3):221-42.

Kerbel RS. (2003). Human tumor xenografts as predictive preclinical models for anticancer drug activity in humans: better than commonly perceived-but they can be improved. *Cancer Biol Ther.* 2(4 Suppl 1):S134-9.

Kim ES and Salgia R. (2009). MET pathway as a therapeutic target. *J Thorac Oncol.* 4(4): 444-7.

Kobayashi S, Boggon TJ, Dayaram T, Jänne PA, Kocher O, Meyerson M, Johnson BE, Eck MJ, Tenen DG, Halmos B. (2005). EGFR mutation and resistance of non-small-cell lung cancer to gefitinib. *N Engl J Med.* 352:786–792.

Kohl NE, Omer CA, Conner MW, Anthony NJ, Davide JP, deSolms SJ, Giuliani EA, Gomez RP, Graham SL, Hamilton K, Handt LK, Hartman GE, Koblan KS, Kral AM, Miller PJ, Mosser SD, O'Neil TJ, Rands E, Schaber MD, Gibbs JB, Oliff A. (1995). Inhibition of farnesyltransferase induces regression of mammary and salivary carcinomas in ras transgenic mice. *Nat Med.* 1(8):792-797.

Kola I and Landis J. (2004). Can the pharmaceutical industry reduce attrition rates? *Nat Rev Drug Discov.* 3(8):711-5.

Kranenburg O. (2005). The KRAS oncogene: past, present, and future. *Biochim. Biophys. Acta.* 1756: 81-82.

Kulke MH, Demetri GD, Sharpless NE, Ryan DP, Shivdasani R, Clark JS, Spiegelman BM, Kim H, Mayer RJ, Fuchs CS. (2002). A phase II study of troglitazone, an activator of the PPARgamma receptor, in patients with chemotherapy-resistant metastatic colorectal cancer. *Cancer J.* 8(5):395-9.

Kung HC, Hoyert D, Xu J, and Murphy SL. (2008). Deaths: Final Data for 2005. *National Vital Statistics Reports.* 56(10):5.

Lambert PF, Pan H, Pitot HC, Liem A, Jackson M, Griep AE. (1993). Epidermal cancer associated with expression of human papillomavirus type 16 E6 and E7 oncogenes in the skin of transgenic mice. *Proc Natl Acad Sci USA.* 90(12):5583-7.

Le Y and Sauer B. (2001). Conditional Gene Knockout Using Cre Recombinase. *Molecular Biotechnology.* 17: 269-275.

Lynch TJ, Bell DW, Sordella R, Gurubhagavatula S, Okimoto RA, Brannigan BW, Harris PL, Haserlat SM, Supko JG, Haluska FG, Louis DN, Christiani DC, Settleman J, Haber DA. (2004). Activating mutations in the epidermal growth factor receptor underlying responsiveness of non-small-cell lung cancer to gefitinib. *N Engl J Med* 350:2129-2139.

Maglione JE, McGoldrick ET, Young LJ, Namba R, Gregg JP, Liu L, Moghanaki D, Ellies LG, Borowsky AD, Cardiff RD, MacLeod CL. (2004). Polyomavirus middle T-induced mammary intraepithelial neoplasia outgrowths: single origin, divergent evolution, and multiple outcomes. *Mol Cancer Ther.* 3(8):941-53.

Maguire HC Jr and Greene MI. (1989). The neu (c-erbB-2) oncogene. *Semin Oncol.*16(2):148-55.

Malkinson AM. (1998). Molecular comparison of human and mouse pulmonary adenocarcinomas. *Exp Lung Res.* 24(4):541-55.

Mangues R, Corral T, Kohl NE, Symmans WF, Lu S, Malumbres M, Gibbs JB, Oliff A, Pellicer A. (1998). Antitumor effect of a farnesyl protein transferase inhibitor in mammary and lymphoid tumors overexpressing N-Ras in transgenic mice. *Cancer Res.* 58(6):1253-1259.

Marino S, Vooijs M, van der Gulden H, Jonker J, Berns A. (2000). Induction of medulloblastomas in p53-null mutant mice by somatic inactivation of Rb in the external granular layer cells of the cerebellum. *Genes Dev.* 14: 994-1004.

Marty M, Cognetti F, Maraninchi D, Snyder R, Mauriac L, Tubiana-Hulin M, Chan S, Grimes D, Antón A, Lluch A, Kennedy J, O'Byrne K, Conte P, Green M, Ward C, Mayne K, Extra JM. (2005). Randomized phase II trial of the efficacy and safety of trastuzumab combined with docetaxel in patients with human epidermal growth factor receptor 2-positive metastatic breast cancer administered as first-line treatment: the M77001 study group. *J Clin Oncol.* 23(19):4265-74.

McLemore MR. (2006). Gardasil: Introducing the new human papillomavirus vaccine. *Clin J Oncol Nurs.* 10(5):559-60.

Mendola CE, Backer JM. (1990). Lovastatin blocks N-ras oncogene-induced neuronal differentiation. *Cell Growth Differ.* 1(10):499-502.

Michel A, Kopp-Schneider A, Zentgraf H, Gruber AD, de Villiers EM. (2006). E6/E7 expression of human papillomavirus type 20 (HPV-20) and HPV-27 influences proliferation and differentiation of the skin in UV-irradiated SKH-hr1 transgenic mice. *J Virol.* 80(22):11153-64.

Monks A, Scudiero D, Skehan P, Shoemaker R, Paull K, Vistica D, Hose C, Langley J, Cronise P, Vaigro-Wolff A, Gray-Goodrich M, Campbell H, Mayo J, Boyd M. (1991). Feasibility of a high-flux anticancer drug screen using a diverse panel of cultured human tumor cell lines. *J Natl Cancer Inst.* 83(11):757-66.

Morita S, Okamoto I, Kobayashi K, Yamazaki K, Asahina H, Inoue A, Hagiwara K, Sunaga N, Yanagitani N, Hida T, Yoshida K, Hirashima T, Yasumoto K, Sugio K, Mitsudomi T, Fukuoka M, Nukiwa T. (2009). Combined survival analysis of prospective clinical trials of gefitinib for non-small cell lung cancer with EGFR mutations. *Clin Cancer Res.* 15(13):4493-8.

Murgo AJ, Kummar S, Rubinstein L, Gutierrez M, Collins J, Kinders R, Parchment RE, Ji J, Steinberg SM, Yang SX, Hollingshead M, Chen A, Helman L, Wiltrout R,

Tomaszewski JE, Doroshow JH. (2008). Designing phase 0 cancer clinical trials. *Clin Cancer Res.* 14(12):3675-82.

Nagy A and Mar L. (2001). Creation and Use of a Cre Recombinase Transgenic Database. *Methods Mol Biol* 158:95-106. Database available from:
<http://nagy.mshri.on.ca/cre/index.php>

Nanda R. (2007). Targeting the human epidermal growth factor receptor 2 (HER2) in the treatment of breast cancer: recent advances and future directions. *Rev Recent Clin Trials.* 2(2):111-6.

Nelson DR, Zeldin DC, Hoffman SM, Maltais LJ, Wain HM, Nebert DW. (2004). Comparison of cytochrome P450 (CYP) genes from the mouse and human genomes, including nomenclature recommendations for genes, pseudogenes and alternative-splice variants. *Pharmacogenetics.* 14(1):1-18.

Ohashi K, Takigawa N, Osawa M, Ichihara E, Takeda H, Kubo T, Hirano S, Yoshino T, Takata M, Tanimoto M, Kiura K. (2009). Chemopreventive Effects of Gefitinib on Nonsmoking-Related Lung Tumorigenesis in Activating Epidermal Growth Factor Receptor Transgenic Mice. *Cancer Res.* 69(17):7088-7095.

Omer CA, Chen Z, Diehl RE, Conner MW, Chen HY, Trumbauer ME, Gopal-Truter S, Seeburger G, Bhimnathwala H, Abrams MT, Davide JP, Ellis MS, Gibbs JB, et al. (2000). Mouse mammary tumor virus-Ki-rasB transgenic mice develop mammary carcinomas that can be growth-inhibited by a farnesyl:protein transferase inhibitor. *Cancer Res.* 60(10):2680-2688.

Ornitz DM, Palmiter RD, Messing A, Hammer RE, Pinkert CA, Brinster RL. (1985). Elastase I promoter directs expression of human growth hormone and SV40 T antigen genes to pancreatic acinar cells in transgenic mice. *Cold Spring Harb Symp Quant Biol.* 50:399-409.

Paez JG, Jänne PA, Lee JC, Tracy S, Greulich H, Gabriel S, Herman P, Kaye FJ, Lindeman N, Boggon TJ, Naoki K, Sasaki H, Fujii Y, Eck MJ, Sellers WR, Johnson BE, Meyerson M. (2004). EGFR mutations in lung cancer: correlation with clinical response to gefitinib therapy. *Science.* 304(5676):1497-500.

Palmiter RD, Chen HY, Messing A, Brinster RL. (1985). SV40 enhancer and large-T antigen are instrumental in development of choroid plexus tumours in transgenic mice. *Nature.* 316(6027):457-60.

Palmiter RD, Brinster RL. (1986). Germ-line transformation of mice. *Annu Rev Genet.* 20:465-99.

Pao W, Miller VA, Politi KA, Riely GJ, Somwar R, Zakowski MF, Kris MG, Varmus H. (2005). Acquired resistance of lung adenocarcinomas to gefitinib or erlotinib is associated with a second mutation in the EGFR kinase domain. *PLoS Med.* 2(3):e73.

Politi K, Zakowski MF, Fan PD, Schonfeld EA, Pao W, Varmus HE. (2006). Lung adenocarcinomas induced in mice by mutant EGF receptors found in human lung cancers respond to a tyrosine kinase inhibitor or to down-regulation of the receptors. *Genes Dev.* 20(11):1496-510.

Poole AJ, Li Y, Kim Y, Lin SC, Lee WH, Lee EY. (2006). Prevention of Brca1-mediated mammary tumorigenesis in mice by a progesterone antagonist. *Science.* 314: 1467-1470.

Quaife CJ, Pinkert CA, Ornitz DM, Palmiter RD, Brinster RL (1987). Pancreatic neoplasia induced by ras expression in acinar cells of transgenic mice. *Cell.* 48(6):1023-34.

Rao PN, Freireich EJ, Smith ML, Loo TL. (1979). Cell cycle phase-specific cytotoxicity of the antitumor agent maytansine. *Cancer Res.* 39(8):3152-5.

Remillard S, Rebhun LI, Howie GA, Kupchan SM. (1975). Antimitotic activity of the potent tumor inhibitor maytansine. *Science.* 189(4207):1002-5.

Riely GJ. (2008). Second-generation epidermal growth factor receptor tyrosine kinase inhibitors in non-small cell lung cancer. *J Thorac Oncol.* 3(6 Suppl 2):S146-9.

Robles AI and Varticovski L. (2008). Harnessing genetically engineered mouse models for preclinical testing. *Chem Biol Interact.* 171(2):159-64.

Rowell CA, Kowalczyk JJ, Lewis MD, Garcia AM. (1997). Direct demonstration of geranylgeranylation and farnesylation of Ki-Ras in vivo. *J Biol Chem.* 272 (22):14093-14097.

Saez E, Tontonoz P, Nelson MC, Alvarez JG, Ming UT, Baird SM, Thomazy VA, Evans RM. (1998). Activators of the nuclear receptor PPARgamma enhance colon polyp formation. *Nat Med.* 4(9):1058-61.

Sarraf P, Mueller E, Jones D, King FJ, DeAngelo DJ, Partridge JB, Holden SA, Chen LB, Singer S, Fletcher C, Spiegelman BM. (1998). Differentiation and reversal of malignant changes in colon cancer through PPARgamma. *Nat Med.* 4(9):1046-52.

Schaper ID, Marcuzzi GP, Weissenborn SJ, Kasper HU, Dries V, Smyth N, Fuchs P, Pfister H. (2005). Development of skin tumors in mice transgenic for early genes of human papillomavirus type 8. *Cancer Res.* 65(4):1394-400.

Sequist LV, Martins RG, Spigel D, Grunberg SM, Spira A, Jänne PA, Joshi VA, McCollum D, Evans TL, Muzikansky A, Kuhlmann GL, Han M, Goldberg JS, Settleman J, Iafrate AJ, Engelman JA, Haber DA, Johnson BE, Lynch TJ. (2008). First-line gefitinib in patients with advanced non-small-cell lung cancer harboring somatic EGFR mutations. *J Clin Oncol.* 26(15):2442-9.

Sharpless NE and Depinho RA. (2006). The mighty mouse: genetically engineered mouse models in cancer drug development. *Nat Rev Drug Discov.* 5(9):741-54.

Shepherd FA, Rodrigues Pereira J, Ciuleanu T, Tan EH, Hirsh V, Thongprasert S, Campos D, Maoleekoonpiroj S, Smylie M, Martins R, van Kooten M, Dediu M, Findlay B, Tu D, Johnston D, Bezjak A, Clark G, Santabárbara P, Seymour L; National Cancer Institute of Canada Clinical Trials Group. (2005). Erlotinib in previously treated non-small-cell lung cancer. *N Engl J Med.* 353(2):123-32.

Shimamura T, Li D, Ji H, Haringsma HJ, Liniker E, Borgman CL, Lowell AM, Minami Y, McNamara K, Perera SA, Zaghlul S, Thomas RK, Greulich H, Kobayashi S, Chirieac LR, Padera RF, Kubo S, Takahashi M, Tenen DG, Meyerson M, Wong KK, Shapiro GI. (2008). Hsp90 inhibition suppresses mutant EGFR-T790M signaling and overcomes kinase inhibitor resistance. *Cancer Res.* 68(14):5827-38.

Slamon DJ, Leyland-Jones B, Shak S, Fuchs H, Paton V, Bajamonde A, Fleming T, Eiermann W, Wolter J, Pegram M, Baselga J, Norton L. (2001). Use of chemotherapy plus a monoclonal antibody against HER2 for metastatic breast cancer that overexpresses HER2. *N Engl J Med.* 2001 Mar 15; 344(11):783-92.

Sos ML, Michel K, Zander T, Weiss J, Frommolt P, Peifer M, Li D, Ullrich R, Koker M, Fischer F, Shimamura T, Rauh D, Mermel C, Fischer S, Stückrath I, Heynck S, et al. (2009). Predicting drug susceptibility of non-small cell lung cancers based on genetic lesions. *J Clin Invest.* 119(6):1727-40.

Sprengel R, Hasan MT. (2007). Tetracycline-controlled genetic switches. *Handb Exp Pharmacol.* (178):49-72.

Stewart TA, Pattengale PK, Leder P. (1984). Spontaneous mammary adenocarcinomas in transgenic mice that carry and express MTV/myc fusion genes. *Cell.* 38(3):627-37.

Strasser A, Harris AW, Bath ML, Cory S. (1990). Novel primitive lymphoid tumours induced in transgenic mice by cooperation between myc and bcl-2. *Nature.* 348(6299):331-3.

Sun J, Qian Y, Hamilton AD, Sebti SM. (1998). Both farnesyltransferase and geranylgeranyltransferase I inhibitors are required for inhibition of oncogenic K-Ras prenylation but each alone is sufficient to suppress human tumor growth in nude mouse xenografts. *Oncogene.* 16(11):1467-1473.

Syrjänen S. (2005). Human papillomavirus (HPV) in head and neck cancer. *J Clin Virol.* 32 Suppl 1:S59-66.

Trotman LC, Niki M, Dotan ZA, Koutcher JA, Di Cristofano A, Xiao A, Khoo AS, Roy-Burman P, Greenberg NM, Van Dyke T, Cordon-Cardo C, Pandolfi PP. (2003). Pten dose dictates cancer progression in the prostate. *PLoS Biol.* 1(3):E59.

Varticovski L, Hollingshead MG, Robles AI, Wu X, Cherry J, Munroe DJ, Lukes L, Anver MR, Carter JP, Borgel SD, Stotler H, Bonomi CA, Nunez NP, Hursting SD, Qiao W, Deng CX, Green JE, Hunter KW, Merlino G, Steeg PS, Wakefield LM, Barrett JC. (2007). Accelerated preclinical testing using transplanted tumors from genetically engineered mouse breast cancer models. *Clin Cancer Res.* 13(7):2168-77.

Ventura A, Kirsch DG, McLaughlin ME, Tuveson DA, Grimm J, Lintault L, Newman J, Reczek EE, Weissleder R, Jacks T. (2007). Restoration of p53 function leads to tumour regression in vivo. *Nature.* 445(7128):661-5.

Wang S, Gao J, Lei Q, Rozengurt N, Pritchard C, Jiao J, Thomas GV, Li G, Roy-Burman P, Nelson PS, Liu X, Wu H. (2003). Prostate-specific deletion of the murine Pten tumor suppressor gene leads to metastatic prostate cancer. *Cancer Cell.* 4(3):209-21.

Weinstein IB. (2002). Addiction to oncogenes--the Achilles heal of cancer. *Science.* 297(5578): 63-4.

Winslow MM, Dayton TL, Verhaak RG, Kim-Kiselak C, Snyder EL, Feldser DM, Hubbard DD, Dupage MJ, Whittaker CA, Hoersch S, Yoon S, Crowley D, Bronson RT, Chiang DY, Meyerson M, Jacks T. (2011). Suppression of lung adenocarcinoma progression by Nkx2-1. *Nature.* 473(7345):101-4.

Yang CH, Yu CJ, Shih JY, Chang YC, Hu FC, Tsai MC, Chen KY, Lin ZZ, Huang CJ, Shun CT, Huang CL, Bean J, Cheng AL, Pao W, Yang PC. (2008). Specific EGFR mutations predict treatment outcome of stage IIIB/IV patients with chemotherapy-naive non-small-cell lung cancer receiving first-line gefitinib monotherapy. *J Clin Oncol.* 26(16):2745-53.

Yun CH, Mengwasser KE, Toms AV, Woo MS, Greulich H, Wong KK, Meyerson M, Eck MJ. (2008). The T790M mutation in EGFR kinase causes drug resistance by increasing the affinity for ATP. *Proc Natl Acad Sci USA.* 105(6):2070-5.

Zenker M, Lehmann K, Schulz AL, Barth H, Hansmann D, Koenig R, Korinthenberg R, Kreiss-Nachtsheim M, Meinecke P, Morlot S, Mundlos S, Quante AS, Raskin S, Schnabel D, Wehner LE, Kratz CP, Horn D, Kutsche K. (2007). Expansion of the genotypic and phenotypic spectrum in patients with KRAS germline mutations. *J. Med. Genet.* 44:131-135.

Zhu K, Hamilton AD, Sebti SM. (2003). Farnesyltransferase inhibitors as anticancer agents: current status. *Curr Opin Investig Drugs.* 4(12):1428-35.

7

Critical Human Hepatocyte-Based *In Vitro* Assays for the Evaluation of Adverse Drug Effects

Albert P. Li

In Vitro ADMET Laboratories LLC and
Advanced Pharmaceutical Sciences Inc., Columbia, MD
USA

1. Introduction

A major challenge in drug development is to accurately estimate human adverse drug effects to allow the selection and advancement of drug candidates with the best safety profile for further development. Due to species differences, safety data obtained with the routine in vivo studies with nonhuman laboratory animals do not always correctly predict human outcome. Human liver-derived systems, especially human hepatocytes, represent physiologically-relevant experimental systems for the evaluation of human adverse drug effects. The assays developed with human-based in vitro experimental systems for the assessment of two major adverse drug effects: drug-drug interactions and drug toxicity can be used routinely during drug development to select and optimize drug candidates to enhance the probability of clinical success.

2. Current challenges in drug development

Efficacy and safety are two co-dependent requirements for successful drug development – clinical failure will result if the drug candidate possesses only one of these two properties. For the past 50 years, drug candidates are evaluated for pharmacological and safety properties using in vivo animal models. It is now known that this paradigm, namely, prediction of human drug properties with animals in vivo, is no longer valid. DiMassi et al (2003)[1] has estimated that for R&D initiated in 2001 with approval 12 years later (based on the average time required for approval), the out-of-pocket cost for a single approved drug is estimated to be U. S. $ 970 million, equivalent to a capitalized cost of U. S. $ 1.9 billion. Frequent clinical trial failure, with lack of efficacy and the occurrence of unexpected adverse drug effects as major reasons, accounts for astronomical time and costs involved in the development of a successful drug. The most recent published estimation of the clinical approval success rate for investigational drugs is 16% [2]. Furthermore, marketed drugs are frequently withdrawn or have their use limited due to adverse effects, with dire consequences to the welfare of the patients and the financial status of the drug manufacturers [3].

3. Overcoming species-species differences

True advancement in the efficiency of drug development can only be made if one accepts that, due to species differences, data from nonhuman laboratory animals do not always predict human drug properties. As in vivo experimentation with humans in vivo during preclinical phases is neither practical nor ethical, surrogates for humans in vivo need to be applied. Experimental models with human tissues and human cells represent practical and relevant surrogates.

A major breakthrough in the acceptance of the reliability of in vitro human-based system in the prediction of human drug properties is the advancement of human-based drug metabolism systems. Human liver fractions (e.g. human liver microsomes), human hepatocytes, and cDNA-derived human drug metabolizing enzymes have been found to provide useful information for the prediction of human metabolism in vivo. These systems are now used routinely for the evaluation of drug metabolism and drug-drug interaction potential of drug candidate in various phases of drug development [4, 5], with the approaches fully endorsed by U. S. FDA [6]. It is interesting to note that the application of in vitro drug metabolism technologies using human-based experimental systems has been attributed to the removal of pharmacokinetics as a major reason for clinical trial failure.

The success in the application of in vitro drug metabolism systems, in combination with data from relevant in vivo animal models, in the prediction of human metabolism suggest that the same approach will also be successful for safety evaluation [7, 8]. Based on the premise that the inability to accurately predict human drug toxicity is due to species-species differences, i. e., there are human-specific drug properties that cannot be revealed by nonhuman animal studies, a safety evaluation strategy is proposed here for the preclinical evaluation of human drug toxicity:

1. Application of **human**-based in vitro systems to provide human-specific toxicity data;
2. Select a relevant animal species to develop **in vivo** parameters;
3. Predict **human in vivo** drug toxicity via a combination of human-specific information obtained in vitro, and in vivo parameters obtained from nonhuman animals in vivo.

Success of this In Vitro-In Vivo Strategy (IVIVS) requires the development of in vitro experimental systems with human-specific properties to cover the key adverse drug effects in humans, and a vigorous set of parameters defining the relevant nonhuman animal species.

4. Human hepatocytes as a key in vitro experimental system for the evaluation of human-specific drug properties

The liver is a key determinant of drug properties. It is a major organ for drug metabolism, and is often a target for drug toxicity [9,10]. Hepatocytes or liver parenchymal cells are the cells in the liver responsible for drug metabolism and are the target cells for hepatotoxic drugs. Isolated hepatocytes therefore represent the most physiologically-relevant experimental system for the evaluation of hepatic drug metabolism and hepatotoxicity [11-13] for the following reasons:

1. Human xenobiotic metabolism: Fresh isolates or cryopreserved fresh isolates of human hepatocytes are known to contain most, if not all, of the in vivo hepatic xenobiotic metabolism capacity [12].

2.   Human target cells: The hepatocytes are the cells in the human liver that are damaged by hepatotoxicants, leading ultimately to liver failure [14,15].

3.   Endpoints: Myriad of toxicological endpoints allowing measurements of necrosis, apoptosis, nuclear receptor interactions, P450 functions, transporter functions etc. have been developed in hepatocytes for the evaluation of adverse drug properties[15,16].

In the past, the use of human hepatocytes has been severely limited by their availability. This limitation has been overcome in the past decade due to advances in the procurement of human livers for research, and the commercial availability of isolated human hepatocytes. The application of human hepatocytes in drug metabolism studies is greatly aided by the successful cryopreservation of human hepatocytes to retain drug metabolism activities [12, 13, 17]. Recently, the usefulness of cryopreserved human hepatocytes is further extended through the development of technologies to cryopreserve human hepatocytes to retain their ability to be cultured as attached cultures (plateable cryopreserved hepatocytes) which can be used for longer term studies such as enzyme induction studies [12].

Cryopreserved human hepatocytes have several advantages over the use of freshly isolated cells:

1.   Experimentation can be readily scheduled;

2.   There are little or no deleterious effects of cryopreservation on key hepatocyte properties;

3.   Repeat of experimentation can be performed at different times or by different laboratories with cells from the same donor;

4.   The hepatocytes can be pre-characterized for properties relevant to a specific study before they are used for experimentation;

5.   Hepatocytes from multiple donor can be used in the same study.

5. Critical assays for the evaluation of adverse drug effects

Two adverse drug effects are responsible for clinical failures and drug withdrawal: drug-drug interactions and drug toxicity. Below are the critical assays for these adverse drug effects. In this chapter, the overall scientific concepts behind these assays and the general approaches used in the assays are described.

6. Critical assays for drug-drug interactions

Metabolic drug-drug interaction results from the alteration of the metabolic clearance of one drug by a co-administered drug. There are two major pathways of metabolic drug-drug interactions:

Inhibitory drug-drug interaction: When one drug inhibits the drug metabolism enzyme responsible for the metabolism of a co-administered drug, the result is a decreased metabolic clearance of the affected drug, resulting in a higher than desired systemic burden. For drugs with a narrow therapeutic index, this may lead to serious toxicological concerns. Most fatal drug-drug interactions are due to inhibitory drug-drug interactions.

Inductive drug-drug interactions: Drug-drug interactions can also be a result of the acceleration of the metabolism of a drug by a co-administered drug. Acceleration of metabolism is usually due to the induction of the gene expression, leading to higher rates of protein synthesis and therefore higher cellular content of the induced drug-metabolizing enzyme and a higher rate of metabolism of the substrates of the induced enzyme. Inductive drug-drug interactions can lead to a higher metabolic clearance of the affected drug, leading to a decrease in plasma concentration and loss of efficacy. Inductive drug-drug interactions can also lead to a higher systemic burden of metabolites, which, if toxic, may lead to safety concerns.

Due to the realization that it is physically impossible to evaluate empirically the possible interaction between one drug and all marketed drugs, and that most drug-metabolizing enzyme pathways are well-defined, a mechanism-based approach is used for the evaluation of drug-drug interaction potential of a new drug or drug candidate [18-20], This mechanistic-based approach is endorsed and required by the U. S. FDA (www.fda.Gov/cber /gdlns/interactstud.htm) for new drug applications. The approach consists of the following major studies:

1. Metabolic phenotyping: The major enzymes involved in the biotransformation of the drug candidate are identified. The major emphasis in the past has been on phase 1 oxidation pathways and on P450 isoforms. Elucidation of enzyme pathways involved in the biotransformation of a drug candidate will allow the identification of potential drug-drug interactions with drugs that are known modifiers (inhibitors and inducers) of the pathways.

    a. Metabolite identification: Structural identification of the metabolites allow one to deduce the major pathways of metabolism. Identification of

        i.   Experimental systems: Human liver homogenate 9000 x g supernatant (S9); human liver microsomes (HLM); hepatocytes

        ii. General incubation conditions:

        1. S9 or HLM: 0.25 to 1.0 mg protein/mL in 0.1 M phosphate buffer at pH 7.4 containing NADPH or NADPH regenerating system (phase 1 oxidation); uridine 5'-diphospho-glucuronic acid (UDPGA; cofactor for glucuronidation) and 3'-phosphoadenosine 5'- phosphosulfate (PAPS; cofactor for sulfation).

        2. Hepatocytes: 0.5 to 1.0 million cells/mL in Isotonic buffer (e.g. Krebs-Hensleit Buffer) maintained at pH 7.2.

        3. Temperature: 37 deg. C

        4. Compound concentration: Generally 10 uM

        5. Time: Multiple time points up to 30 minutes (HLM); 2 hrs (hepatocytes in suspension); 24 hrs. (hepatocytes in monolayer culture)

        iii. Metabolite identification: HPLC-MS/MS is the most commonly used approach for the initial identification of the metabolites. NMR is used for definitive structural identification.

    b. Major pathway identification: Chemical inhibitors are used to identify of the major oxidative pathways involved in the formation of the metabolites. Inhibition of metabolism of the parent compound, as indicated by metabolic stability or decreased formation of metabolites, would suggest that the participation of the pathway in the metabolism of the compound. Examples of inhibitors for the major pathways are as follows:

        i.   P450 inhibition: 1-aminobenzotriazole (S9; HLM; hepatocytes)

        ii. MAO inhibitors: pargyline (S9)

        iii. FMO inhibitiors: 45 deg. C inactivation (S9; HLM).

    c. P450 isoform identification:

    i.   Experimental system: HLM or cDNA-P450 isoforms

    ii.   Incubation with HLM in the presence of isoform-selective inhibitors or individual cDNA-P450 isoforms to determine pathway responsible for metabolism. Inhibition of metabolism by an inhibitor of a specific isoform (Table 1) with corroborative data using the identified cDNA-P450 isoform would allow the identification of the isoform for the metabolism of the compound in question.

  d.   Evaluation of inhibitory potential for drug-metabolizing enzymes: The drug candidate will be evaluated for its ability to inhibit known drug metabolizing enzymes, with emphasis on the P450 isoforms. The incubation conditions are similar to that described above for metabolite identification, using substrates that are selective for the pathways in question (Table 1).

  e.   Evaluation of induction potential for drug metabolizing enzymes: The drug candidate will be evaluated for its ability to induce known drug metabolizing enzymes. The inducible P450 isoforms: CYP1A, 2B and 3A are the ones required by U. S. FDA. Human hepatocytes are considered the "gold standard" for induction studies, with cryopreserved hepatocytes that can be cultured after thawing and have been characterized to be responsive to prototypical inducers as the preferred system. As of this writing, virtually all known inducers of P450 isoforms in vivo are inducers in human hepatocytes in vitro (Table 1) [12]. Experimental evaluation of enzyme induction involves the treatment of human hepatocytes for several days with the test article followed by evaluation of enzyme activities using P450 isoform-specific substrates [20].

The general experimental conditions are as follows:

    i.   Experimental system: Primary cultured human hepatocytes

    ii.   Culturing condition: Matrigel-collagen sandwich (requirement: >80% confluent cultures).

    iii.   Treatment regiment: Culturing of hepatocytes for 2 days followed by 3 days of treatment

    iv.   Endpoints: Quantification of CYP1A2, 2B6 and 3A4 gene expression by RT-PCR as well as activities using isoform-specific substrates (Table 1).

7. Higher throughput human hepatocyte-based drug-drug interaction studies

Of the multiple P450 isoforms, CYP3A4 is the most abundant of the isoforms in the human liver. CYP3A4 has been found to be responsible for the metabolism of a large variety of exogenous and endogenous substrates [21, 22]. In drug development, there is a need to evaluate the inhibitory and inductive potential of drug candidates towards CYP3A4 to estimate their drug-drug interaction potential with the myriad drugs that are substrates of this important P450 isoform [23-25]. In our laboratory, we have developed cost- and time-effective higher throughput screening assays for the evaluation of drug-drug interaction potential of drug candidates involving CYP3A4. The assays are as follows:

1.   384-well CYP3A4 inhibition assay [26];

2.   96-well time-dependent CYP3A4 inhibition assay [27];

3.   96-well CYP3A4 induction assay [26].

The throughput of the assays are increased via the use of the following technologies:

1. Cryopreserved human hepatocytes cultured in micro-well cell culture plates: The properties and advantages of cryopreserved human hepatocytes have been discussed earlier. The use of micr-owell (96 and 384 well plates) allows the ease of sample organization, decreased cost of cells and reagents, and allows the use of automation.

2. Luciferin-IPA as CYP3A4 substrate: Luciferin-IPA is metabolized to luciferin specifically by CYP3A4. The use of this substrate allows CYP3A4 activity to be quantified using a plate-reader, thereby eliminating the need for the time-consuming and costly LC/MS assays that are used with conventional substrates.

P450 Isoforms	Substrates	Inhibitors	Inducers
CYP1A2	7-ethoxyresorufin dealkylation; Phenacetin-O-deethylation	Furafylline; a-naphthoflavone	3-methylcholanthrene; omeprazole
CYP2A6	Courmarin 7-hydroxylation	Tranylcypromine; methoxsalen	Dexamethasone
CYP2B6	Buproprion hydroxylation	Ticlopidine; clopidogrel	Phenobarbital; phenytoin
CYP2C8	Taxol 6-hydroxylation	Quercetin	Rifampin
CYP2C9	Tolbutamide methyl-hydroxylation	Sulphenazole	Rifampin
CYP2C19	S-mephenytoin 4'-hydroxylation	Omeprazole	Rifampin
CYP2D6	Dextromethorphan O-demethylation	Quinidine	none
CYP2E1	Chloroxazone 6-hydroxylation	Diethyldithiocarbamide	none
CYP3A4/5	Midazolam 1-hydroxylation; testosterone 6b-hydroxylation; luciferin-IPA dealkylation	Ketoconazole; itraconazole; troleandomycin; verapamil	Rifampin; phenobarbital; phenytoin; troglitazone

Table 1. Model P450 isoform-selective substrates, inhibitors, and inducers. These compounds can be used for pathway identification (inhibitors); evaluation of isoform-selective inhibition (substrates); and as positive controls for the evaluation of P450 induction (inducers).

8. 384 well CYP3A inhibition assay with intact human hepatocytes

Evaluation of P450 inhibition is traditionally performed with liver microsomes and recombinant CYP enzymes [28, 29]. Intact hepatocytes represent an additional experimental system that may provide useful information to improve the accuracy of the prediction of in vivo effects. A chemical, for instance, may be metabolized by non-CYP pathways to a metabolite that is a potent P450 inhibitor and therefore would be inhibitory in hepatocytes but not in microsomes or recombinant CYP enzymes. Gemfibrozil, for instance, requires glucuronidation for its CYP2C8 inhibitory effects and is found to be a potent CYP2C8 inhibitor in hepatocytes but not in liver microsomes nor recombinant CYP2C8[30]. Hepatocytes can also be used for the modeling of differential inhibitor distribution between plasma and intracellular compartments. Lu et al. reported the use of hepatocytes suspended in 100% human plasma to accurately predict CYP3A4 inhibitory effects of several CYP3A inhibitors in vivo [31]. The presence of active transporters in human hepatocytes, including cryopreserved hepatocytes, also suggests that an inhibitor may be actively accumulated inside the cells, leading to substantially higher concentration and a correspondingly higher inhibitory effect which would not be observed using cell free systems [32, 33].

We have previously introduced the use of human hepatocytes in P450 inhibition studies [20, 34, 35]. In the HTS human hepatocyte CYP3A4 inhibition assay described here, 384-well plates were used to reduce the quantity of hepatocytes, reagents, as well as the chemical to be evaluated[26]. The use of LIPA as CYP3A4 substrate substantially enhances the efficiency of the assay, as its metabolism can be quantified based of luminescence using a plate reader [35], thereby eliminating the need for HPLC and mass spectrometry that are routinely required with conventional substrates such as testosterone and midazolam. The use of robotics allowed rapid and accurate delivery of relatively small volumes of reagents into the 384 well plates. The accuracy of the assay is demonstrated by the relatively low coefficient of variation (standard deviations <10% of mean values) of the results.

A homogenous (addition assay) has been developed in our laboratory using cryopreserved human hepatocytes cultured in 384 well plates. An automated workstation is used for the performance of the assay. The workstation is programmed to perform serial dilutions of the model inhibitors and for the initiation of the assay. White opaque 384-well plates are used. The workstation is programmed to add into each of the wells of the 384-well plates 10 uL of hepatocytes (containing 10,000 cells) and 10 uL of Hepatocyte Metabolism Medium containing either solvent (0.1% v/v of acetonitrile) or P450 inhibitors at the designated concentrations (at 3X of the designated concentrations). The assay is initiated by the addition of 10 uL of 3 uM LIPA (final concentration 1 uM). The plates are returned to a cell culture incubator maintained at 37 deg. C, in a highly humidified atmosphere of 95% air and 5% carbon dioxide. After an incubation period of 120 minutes, the plates are returned to the workstation for the addition of 10 uL of Luciferin Detection Reagent. Luminescence is quantified using a multichannel plate reader.

Representative results of the application of this HTS assay to evaluate CYP3A4 inhibitory potential of drug substances, using model CYP3A4 inhibitors, are shown in Fig. 1.

9. 96-well time-dependent inhibition assay for CYP3A4 in human hepatocytes

In terms of P450 inhibition, time-dependent inhibition (TDI) or mechanism-based P450 inhibition is of particular concern. In TDI, the inactivated P450 needs to be replaced by newly synthesized proteins to return to its normal activity. After cessation of administration with the TDI inhibitor, the patient would continue to have decreased drug metabolizing capacity before the inactivated enzymes are fully replaced [23, 36].

While TDI is generally studied using liver microsomes or recombinant CYP [37, 38], there are substantial efforts in the evaluation of this important mechanism of drug-drug interaction in human hepatocytes [39, 40]. Human hepatocytes, because of the intact plasma membrane, complete and uninterrupted drug metabolism enzymes and cofactors, represent a desirable in vitro experimental system for the evaluation of human drug properties.

Traditionally, TDI studies with hepatocytes utilize suspension cultures [40]. The use of hepatocytes in suspension culture is a common practice with cryopreserved cells as most preparations of cryopreserved hepatocytes would have compromised ability to be cultured as monolayer cultures. Due to our success in cryopreservation of human hepatocytes to retain their ability to be cultured, a convenient and quantitative approach for the evaluation of TDI using monolayer cultures of plateable cryopreserved human hepatocytes has been developed in our laboratory[41].

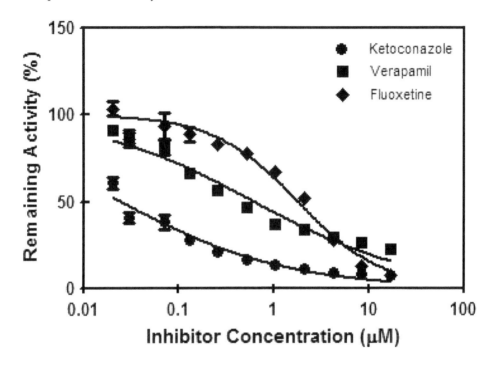

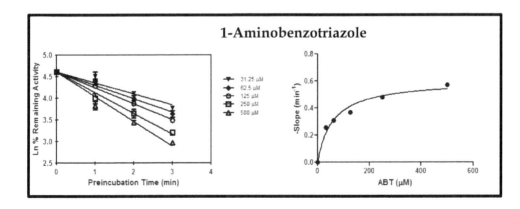

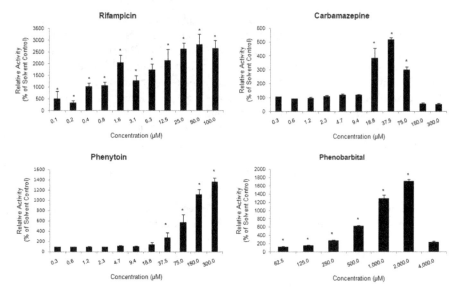

Fig. 1. Examples of the application of the higher throughput hepatocyte assays in the evaluation of CYP3A4 inhibition (top panel), time-dependent CYP3A4 inhibition (middle panel), and CYP3A4 induction. For the CYP3A4 inhibition assay, dose-dependent inhibition was observed for the three model inhibitors, ketoconazole, verapamil, and fluoxetine (top panel). The model time-dependent inhibitor, 1-aminobenzotriazole, yielded time-dependent and dose-dependent inhibition (left figure, middle panel). A plot of the slop of the time-dependent decrease in activity versus inhibitor concentration yielded the classical saturation curve (right figure, middle panel) which can be used to calculate the time-dependent inhibition enzyme kinetic constants kinact and KI. The model CYP3A4 inducers rifampin, carbamazepine, phenytoin and phenobarbital yielded dose dependent induction of CYP3A4 activity (bottom panel). From Li[35]; Doshi and Li[26]; and Li and Doshi[27].

In this assay, the cryopreserved human hepatocytes are thawed from cryopreservation using Cryopreserved Hepatocytes Recovery Medium and plated at 50,000 cells per well in 96-well collagen coated plates in Cryopreserved Hepatocytes Plating Medium at a volume of 100 uL per well. The cells are cultured for 4 hours in a cell culture incubator maintained at 37 deg. C with a highly humidified atmosphere of 5% carbon dioxide and 95% air. The cells on the day of plating (4 hour cultures) are used for the evaluation of TDI. The plating medium is removed and the cells are washed 3 times with Hepatocyte Metabolism Medium (HMM), followed by the addition of 50 uL of HMM per well. At designated times 50 uL of treatment media consisting of HMM containing 2X concentrated solutions of the inhibitors or medium control is added. At designated periods after treatment media are removed by quickly inverting the 96-well plates on absorbent paper. The cells are washed 5 times with 100 uL of HMM to remove the inhibitors. The cells are incubated at 37 deg. C with 100 uL per well of HMM for a 60 min "washout" period to allow removal of intracellular inhibitors by diffusion to minimize competitive inhibition with CYP3A4 substrate. After the washout period, medium is replaced with that containing 3 uM of the CYP3A4-specific substrate LIPA. After an incubation period of 30 min, 50 uL of the incubated substrate solution from each well is removed and placed into a white 96-well plate. After all the solutions are collected from the various time points, 50 uL of Luciferin Detection Reagent is added to each well containing incubated substrate solution followed by quantification of luminescence using a Wallac Victor-3 plate reader. Luminescence signals are converted to pmoles of luciferin based on a standard curve generated from luciferin. Viability of the hepatocytes after treatment is determined after CYP3A4 activity quantification using cellular ATP as an endpoint using a commercially available ATP kit consisting of lysis buffer and ATP detection reagent.

Results are expressed as % remaining activity, which is calculated as a ratio of the activity in the presence of inhibitors to that of the solvent control using the following equation:

$$\% \text{ Remaining Activity (\%)} = [\text{Normalized Activity (Treatment)}/\text{Normalized Activity (Solvent Control)}] \times 100;$$

whereas activity represents luciferin generated in each well quantified by luminescence normalized by relative activity based on ATP content using the following equations:

$$\text{Normalized Activity} = \text{CYP3A4 Activity}/\text{Relative Viability}$$

$$\text{Relative Viability (\%)} = \text{ATP Content (Treatment)}/\text{ATP Content (Solvent Control)}$$

Enzyme kinetic parameters for TDI are derived as follows: The observed rate of enzyme inactivation (k_{obs}) is determined as the initial slope of the linear regression line of a semi-logarithmic plot of the natural logarithm of remaining activity versus preincubation time. k_{inact} and K_I values are determined based on the double reciprocal Lineweaver-Burk plot ($1/k_{obs}$ versus $1/[I]$, whereas [I] represents inhibitor concentration), where k_{inact} is estimated as the reciprocal of the Y-intercept and K_I as the negative reciprocal of the x-intercept.

Representative results of the application of this HTS assay to evaluate time-dependent CYP3A4 inhibitory potential of drug substances, using the model time-dependent CYP3A4 inhibitor, 1-aminobenzotriazole, are shown in Fig. 1.

10. 96-well CYP3A4 induction assay with human hepatocytes

Enzyme induction is a major mechanism for drug-drug interactions. Induction of a drug metabolizing enzyme by one drug would lead to the enhanced metabolism of co-administered drugs that are substrates of the induced enzyme.

As freshly isolated hepatocytes possess endogenous activities which may be the result of inducers present in the donor's systemic circulation, the isolated hepatocytes are cultured for 2 to 3 days to allow the P450 enzyme activities to return to a basal level. Testing for induction potential is that initiated by treatment of the cultured hepatocytes for 2 to 3 days to allow full expression of the induced enzyme. Induction is generally evaluated by measuring enzyme activity as activity represents the most relevant endpoint for drug-drug interaction. Both freshly isolated and plateable cryopreserved human hepatocytes can be used for the induction study.

In our laboratory, we have developed a higher-throughput P450 induction assay using 96 well plates[26]. The procedures are as follows:

1. Day 0: Plate human hepatocytes (freshly isolated or plateable cryopreserved human hepatocytes) with 50 uL of cell suspension per well, at a cell density of 1 million cells/mL thereby delivering 50,000 cells per well.

2. Day 1: Change medium to cold (4 to 10 deg. C) medium containing 0.25 mg/mL of Matrigel®.
3. Day 2: Change medium to treatment medium containing test articles at the desired concentrations.
4. Day 3, 4, 5: Continue treatment. Medium change is not necessary unless the test article is known to be unstable under the culturing conditions.
5. Day 6: Measure activity (in situ incubation with LIPA) or extraction of RNA for the evaluation of gene expression.

Representative results of the application of this HTS assay to evaluate CYP3A4 induction potential of drug substances, using model CYP3A4 inducers, are shown in Fig. 1.

11. In vitro evaluation of drug toxicity

The current success in the application of human-based in vitro experimental models in the evaluation of drug metabolism and drug-drug interactions paths the way for a similar approach to evaluate drug toxicity, especially human-specific toxic events that cannot be observed in laboratory animals. In vitro toxicity assays are can be applied in various during phases of drug development:

1. **Early screening of intrinsic toxicity:** Cell-based systems are used for rapid screening of drug candidates, especially structural analogs, to allow the selection of less toxic structures for further development. The screening assay can allow logical evaluation of structures responsible for toxicity (toxicophore) which, hopefully, can be separated from structures for pharmacological activity (pharmacophore). Toxicity screening with in vitro systems require only limited amount of test articles, and is rapid and quantitative. Toxicity is most effective when one has an indication for in vivo toxicity (e.g. hepatotoxicity or nephrotoxicity) for a lead molecule, therefore allowing the selection of the most appropriate in vitro system for screening (e.g. hepatocytes for hepatotoxicity and renal proximal tubule cells for nephrotoxicity).
2. **Mechanistic evaluations:** Mechanistic understanding is critical to drug development. It allows a better understanding of human health risks, defines potential risk factors, and evaluates the relationship between efficacy and adverse effects. Mechanistic studies may be performed after adverse effects are observed in nonhuman animals to aid the prediction of human toxicity as well as the development of approaches for a more acceptable replacement. The defined experimental conditions and the availability of reagents and approaches for multiple endpoints of in vitro experimental systems allow one to define the key pathways involved in a toxicology phenomenon.

The preferred human in vitro systems for the evaluation of drug toxicity are primary cells derived from human organs, used within a period that the cells would retain differentiated functions, thereby serving as surrogates of the similar cells in vivo.

Primary cell culture systems, including stem-cell derived differentiated cells representative of the key cell types in each organ, are currently available and the respective organ-specific toxicity:

*   Hepatocytes (hepatotoxicity)
*   Renal proximal tubule epithelial cells (nephrotoxicity)
*   Vascular endothelial cells (vascular toxicity)
*   Neuronal cells, glial cells and astrocytes (neurotoxicity)

- Cardiomyocytes (cardiotoxicity)
- Bone marrow cells (bone marrow toxicity)

12. Overcoming the major deficiencies of in vitro system

An argument routinely raised against the application of in vitro systems in safety evaluation is that toxicity is a complex phenomenon and therefore cannot be adequately modeled by simple in vitro systems such as cell culture assays.

The major deficiencies of in vitro experimental systems can be defined as follows:

1. **Lack of systemic effects.** In vitro experimental systems in general consist of single cell types. Toxic effects are evaluated in the absence of influences from systemic effects that may be critical to drug toxicity. An example is the participation of the immune system in organ toxicity. One hypothesis for idiosyncratic hepatotoxicity, for instance, is the hapten-hypothesis which postulates that liver failure arises from the cytotoxicity of antibodies towards antigens developed between the idiosyncratic drug (or its metabolites) on the plasma membrane of the hepatocytes.

2. **Absence of chronic dosing.** It is generally believe that drug toxicity due to acute cytotoxic events can be studied effectively with in vitro systems. However, toxic effects due to chronic, low-dose treatments may require multiple events that may or may not be obtained with in vitro studies, with cells treated for a relatively short time period (e.g. 24-hours). Long-term treatments (e.g. months to years) of cells in culture is theoretically possible but in practice near impossible. Further, it is extremely difficult to maintain primary cells, the preferred cell system, in a differentiated state for a long time period.

For in vitro systems to be useful, one needs to develop experimental approaches to overcome these deficiencies.

13. In vitro experimental model for multiple organ interactions: Integrated discrete multiple organ co-culture (IdMOC)

One major drawback of in vitro system is that each cell type is studied in isolation. In the human body, multiple organ interactions may be critical to drug toxicity. An example of multiple organ interactions is a drug which is firstly metabolized by one organ (e.g. liver) to form metabolites which may enter the general systemic circulation to cause toxicity in a distant organ (e.g. heart).

The multiple organ interaction is not covered by the TACIT approach[8] using a single cell type, as the initiating events may include effects of a toxicant on a nontarget cell. To overcome this deficiency, we have developed the IdMOC (Independent Discrete Multiple Organ Co-culture) system ([42-44]). The IdMOC allows the co-culturing of cells from different organs as physically separated cultures that are interconnected by an overlying medium, akin to the blood circulation connecting the multiple organs in the human body (Fig. 1). The IdMOC models the multiple organ interaction in the whole organism in vivo, allowing the evaluation of organ-specific effects a drug and its metabolites. The IdMOC represents an improved in vitro experimental system for routine screening of ADMET drug properties.

The IdMOC involves the "wells-in-a-well" concept. The typical IdMOC plate consists of a chamber within which are several wells (Fig. 2). Cells of different origins (e.g. from different organs) are initially cultured, each in its specific medium, in the wells. When the cells are established, the wells are flooded with an overlying medium, thereby connecting all the wells. The multiple cell types now can interact via the overlying medium, akin to the multiple organs in a human body interacting via the systemic circulation.

The IdMOC system can be used for the following:

1. Differential cytotoxicity: Evaluation of the toxicity of a substance on different cell types (e.g. cells from different organs) under virtually identical experimental conditions with multiple cell-type interactions. Aflatoxin B1, a know hepatotoxicant in humans in vivo, is shown to have selectively higher cytotoxicity in hepatocytes in the IdMOC co-culture of hepatocytes, renal proximal tubule cells, and small airway epithelial cells.
2. Differential distribution: Evaluation of the differential accumulation/distribution of a substance among multiple cell types. This application is especially useful for the development of cytotoxic anticancer agent with selective affinity towards cancer cells.
3. Multiple organ metabolism: Evaluate the ultimate metabolic fate of a substance upon metabolism by cells representing multiple organs with metabolic functions (e.g. liver, kidney, lung). This application allows the development of metabolite profiling of drugs which are subjected to both hepatic and extrahepatic metabolism.

Evaluate of organ-specific toxicity is illustrated by the treatment of IdMOC with a known hepatotoxicant, aflatoxin B1, in IdMOC with three human primary cell types: hepatocytes, renal proximal tubule epithelial cells, and pulmonary (small airway) epithelial cells. Aflatoxin B1 was found to be significantly more cytotoxic towards human hepatocytes, presumably due to the higher P450 activities of the cells versus the other two cell types (Fig. 3), as it is known that aflatoxin requires P450 metabolism to toxic metabolites to exert its toxicity.

14. Conclusion

Accurate prediction of human adverse drug effects represents a major challenge for drug development. The high rate of clinical failure of drug candidates that have been carefully selected from preclinical studies illustrates clearly that the routine, "classical" approach of preclinical safety evaluation is inadequate. It is argued here that species-species differences in drug toxicity is a major reason – human-specific toxicity, by definition, cannot be predicted with nonhuman laboratory animals. It is proposed here that human in vivo drug toxicity can be predicted using a combination of human-based in vitro experimental systems and appropriate in vivo laboratory animals - the In Vitro-In Vivo Strategy (IVIVS). The success of IVIVS will depend on the selection of appropriate in vitro models. Human-specific drug metabolism, appropriate target cell populations, and relevant endpoints are three key parameters for the selection of an appropriate in vitro model. Human hepatocytes and human liver fractions represent useful appropriate experimental models to evaluate liver specific events such as hepatic metabolism, drug-drug interactions, and hepatotoxicity. Higher throughput screening assays have been developed to allow early screening of human-specific adverse drug effects. IdMOC allows the co-culturing of multiple cell types modeling in vivo multiple organ interactions and thereby represent a more complete in vitro experimental system for the prediction of in vivo drug properties.

It is to be noted that recent research findings have demonstrated that in addition to drug metabolizing enzyme activities, uptake and efflux transporters also play critical roles in the manifestation of adverse drug effects [10, 45]. Human hepatocyte assays for the evaluation of uptake and efflux transporters have been established and are being applied towards drug development [46-50]. These transporter assays, when applied in conjunction with the assays described in this chapter, should aid the selection of the most appropriate drug candidates for further drug development.

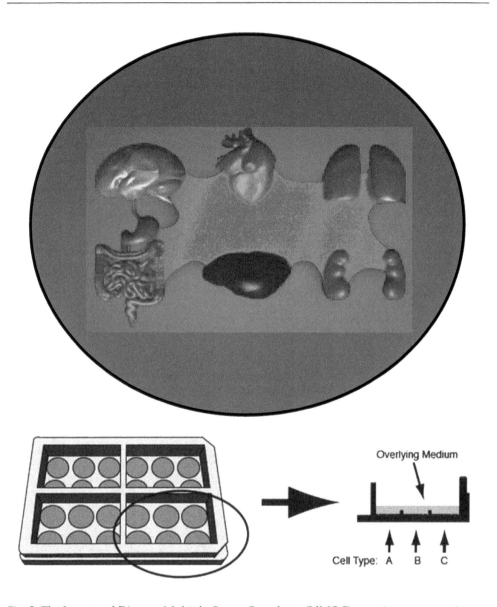

Fig. 2. The Integrated Discrete Multiple Organ Co-culture (IdMOC) experiment system is based on the concept that in the human body consists of multiple organs interacting via the systemic circulation (Top figure). A toxicant may be metabolized by one or more of the organs, and the resulting metabolites may interact with one or more organs via the systemic circulation. This concept is reduced to practice as an IdMOC plate (Lower Figure), with multiple wells within a chamber. Cells from individual organs are cultured physically separated in the wells, with the cells of the multiple organs interconnected via an overlying medium. From Li [43]

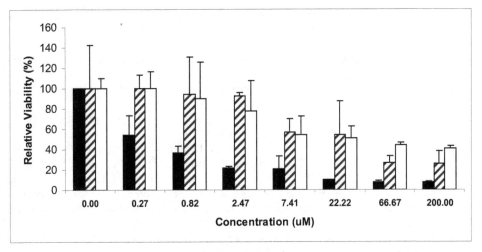

Fig. 3. Application of the Integrated Discrete Multiple Organ Co-culture (IdMOC) experiment system in the evaluation of organ specific toxicity. IdMOC with co-cultures of human hepatocytes (solid bars), renal proximal tubule cells (shaded bars), and small airway epithelial cells (open bars) was used to evaluate the cytotoxicity of the known hepatotoxic agent, aflatoxin B1. While dose-dependent cytotoxicity was observed for all cell types, aflatoxin B1 was significantly more cytotoxic towards human hepatocytes. The results illustrate the application of IdMOC in the evaluation of organ-selective toxicity of drug substances. Other applications of IdMOC include organ-selective drug distribution and integrated multiple organ metabolism.

15. References

[1] DiMasi JA, Hansen RW, Grabowski HG: The price of innovation: new estimates of drug development costs, J Health Econ 2003, 22:151-185

[2] DiMasi JA, Feldman L, Seckler A, Wilson A: Trends in risks associated with new drug development: success rates for investigational drugs, Clin Pharmacol Ther 2010, 87:272-277

[3] Wysowski DK, Swartz L: Adverse drug event surveillance and drug withdrawals in the United States, 1969-2002: the importance of reporting suspected reactions, Arch Intern Med 2005, 165:1363-1369

[4] Li AP, Jurima-Romet M: Overview: pharmacokinetic drug-drug interactions, Adv Pharmacol 1997, 43:1-6

[5] Davit B, Reynolds K, Yuan R, Ajayi F, Conner D, Fadiran E, Gillespie B, Sahajwalla C, Huang SM, Lesko LJ: FDA evaluations using in vitro metabolism to predict and interpret in vivo metabolic drug-drug interactions: impact on labeling, J Clin Pharmacol 1999, 39:899-910

[6] Zhang L, Zhang YD, Zhao P, Huang SM: Predicting drug-drug interactions: an FDA perspective, AAPS J 2009, 11:300-306

[7] MacGregor JT, Collins JM, Sugiyama Y, Tyson CA, Dean J, Smith L, Andersen M, Curren RD, Houston JB, Kadlubar FF, Kedderis GL, Krishnan K, Li AP, Parchment RE,

Thummel K, Tomaszewski JE, Ulrich R, Vickers AE, Wrighton SA: In vitro human tissue models in risk assessment: report of a consensus-building workshop, Toxicol Sci 2001, 59:17-36

[8] Li AP: Human-based in vitro experimental systems for the evaluation of human drug safety, Curr Drug Saf 2007, 2:193-199

[9] Ikeda T: Drug-induced idiosyncratic hepatotoxicity: prevention strategy developed after the troglitazone case, Drug Metab Pharmacokinet 2011, 26:60-70

[10] Assis DN, Navarro VJ: Human drug hepatotoxicity: a contemporary clinical perspective, Expert Opin Drug Metab Toxicol 2009, 5:463-473

[11] Hewitt NJ, Lechon MJ, Houston JB, Hallifax D, Brown HS, Maurel P, Kenna JG, Gustavsson L, Lohmann C, Skonberg C, Guillouzo A, Tuschl G, Li AP, LeCluyse E, Groothuis GM, Hengstler JG: Primary hepatocytes: current understanding of the regulation of metabolic enzymes and transporter proteins, and pharmaceutical practice for the use of hepatocytes in metabolism, enzyme induction, transporter, clearance, and hepatotoxicity studies, Drug Metab Rev 2007, 39:159-234

[12] Li AP: Human hepatocytes: isolation, cryopreservation and applications in drug development, Chem Biol Interact 2007, 168:16-29

[13] Li AP: Human hepatocytes as an effective alternative experimental system for the evaluation of human drug properties: general concepts and assay procedures, ALTEX 2008, 25:33-42

[14] Ulrich RG, Rockett JC, Gibson GG, Pettit SD: Overview of an interlaboratory collaboration on evaluating the effects of model hepatotoxicants on hepatic gene expression, Environ Health Perspect 2004, 112:423-427

[15] Gomez-Lechon MJ, Castell JV, Donato MT: The use of hepatocytes to investigate drug toxicity, Methods Mol Biol 2010, 640:389-415

[16] O'Brien PJ, Chan K, Silber PM: Human and animal hepatocytes in vitro with extrapolation in vivo, Chem Biol Interact 2004, 150:97-114

[17] Loretz LJ, Li AP, Flye MW, Wilson AG: Optimization of cryopreservation procedures for rat and human hepatocytes, Xenobiotica 1989, 19:489-498

[18] Li AP: Preclinical evaluation of drug-drug interactions using human in vitro experimental systems, IDrugs 1998, 1:311-314

[19] Li AP: Primary hepatocyte cultures as an in vitro experimental model for the evaluation of pharmacokinetic drug-drug interactions, Adv Pharmacol 1997, 43:103-130

[20] Li AP: Evaluation of drug metabolism, drug-drug interactions, and in vitro hepatotoxicity with cryopreserved human hepatocytes, Methods Mol Biol 2010, 640:281-294

[21] Li AP, Kaminski DL, Rasmussen A: Substrates of human hepatic cytochrome P450 3A4, Toxicology 1995, 104:1-8

[22] Guengerich FP: Cytochrome P450: what have we learned and what are the future issues?, Drug Metab Rev 2004, 36:159-197

[23] Zhou SF, Xue CC, Yu XQ, Li C, Wang G: Clinically important drug interactions potentially involving mechanism-based inhibition of cytochrome P450 3A4 and the role of therapeutic drug monitoring, Ther Drug Monit 2007, 29:687-710

[24] Flockhart DA, Oesterheld JR: Cytochrome P450-mediated drug interactions, Child Adolesc Psychiatr Clin N Am 2000, 9:43-76

[25] Fujita K: Food-drug interactions via human cytochrome P450 3A (CYP3A), Drug Metabol Drug Interact 2004, 20:195-217

[26] Doshi U, Li AP: Luciferin IPA-Based Higher Throughput Human Hepatocyte Screening Assays for CYP3A4 Inhibition and Induction, J Biomol Screen 2011,

[27] Li AP, Doshi U: Higher Throughput Human Hepatocyte Assays for the Evaluation of Time-Dependent Inhibition of CYP3A4, Drug Metab Lett 2011,

[28] Chauret N, Tremblay N, Lackman RL, Gauthier JY, Silva JM, Marois J, Yergey JA, Nicoll-Griffith DA: Description of a 96-well plate assay to measure cytochrome P4503A inhibition in human liver microsomes using a selective fluorescent probe, Anal Biochem 1999, 276:215-226

[29] Crespi CL, Penman BW: Use of cDNA-expressed human cytochrome P450 enzymes to study potential drug-drug interactions, Adv Pharmacol 1997, 43:171-188

[30] Ogilvie BW, Zhang D, Li W, Rodrigues AD, Gipson AE, Holsapple J, Toren P, Parkinson A: Glucuronidation converts gemfibrozil to a potent, metabolism-dependent inhibitor of CYP2C8: implications for drug-drug interactions, Drug Metab Dispos 2006, 34:191-197

[31] Lu C, Hatsis P, Berg C, Lee FW, Balani SK: Prediction of pharmacokinetic drug-drug interactions using human hepatocyte suspension in plasma and cytochrome P450 phenotypic data. II. In vitro-in vivo correlation with ketoconazole, Drug Metab Dispos 2008, 36:1255-1260

[32] Shitara Y, Li AP, Kato Y, Lu C, Ito K, Itoh T, Sugiyama Y: Function of uptake transporters for taurocholate and estradiol 17beta-D-glucuronide in cryopreserved human hepatocytes, Drug Metab Pharmacokinet 2003, 18:33-41

[33] Maeda K, Kambara M, Tian Y, Hofmann AF, Sugiyama Y: Uptake of ursodeoxycholate and its conjugates by human hepatocytes: role of Na(+)-taurocholate cotransporting polypeptide (NTCP), organic anion transporting polypeptide (OATP) 1B1 (OATP-C), and oatp1B3 (OATP8), Mol Pharm 2006, 3:70-77

[34] Li AP, Lu C, Brent JA, Pham C, Fackett A, Ruegg CE, Silber PM: Cryopreserved human hepatocytes: characterization of drug-metabolizing enzyme activities and applications in higher throughput screening assays for hepatotoxicity, metabolic stability, and drug-drug interaction potential, Chem Biol Interact 1999, 121:17-35

[35] Li AP: Evaluation of luciferin-isopropyl acetal as a CYP3A4 substrate for human hepatocytes: effects of organic solvents, cytochrome P450 (P450) inhibitors, and P450 inducers, Drug Metab Dispos 2009, 37:1598-1603

[36] Zhou ZW, Zhou SF: Application of mechanism-based CYP inhibition for predicting drug-drug interactions, Expert Opin Drug Metab Toxicol 2009, 5:579-605

[37] Wang X, Wang Y, Chunsheng Y, Wang L, Han S: Mechanism-based quantitative structure-phytotoxicity relationships comparative inhibition of substituted phenols on root elongation of Cucumis sativus, Arch Environ Contam Toxicol 2002, 42:29-35

[38] Mori K, Hashimoto H, Takatsu H, Tsuda-Tsukimoto M, Kume T: Cocktail-substrate assay system for mechanism-based inhibition of CYP2C9, CYP2D6, and CYP3A using human liver microsomes at an early stage of drug development, Xenobiotica 2009, 39:415-422

[39] McGinnity DF, Berry AJ, Kenny JR, Grime K, Riley RJ: Evaluation of time-dependent cytochrome P450 inhibition using cultured human hepatocytes, Drug Metab Dispos 2006, 34:1291-1300

[40] Mao J, Mohutsky MA, Harrelson JP, Wrighton SA, Hall SD: Prediction of CYP3A-Mediated Drug-Drug Interactions Using Human Hepatocytes Suspended in Human Plasma, Drug Metab Dispos 2011, 39:591-602

[41] Li AP, Doshi U: Higher Throughput Human Hepatocyte Assays for the Evaluation of Time-Dependent Inhibition of CYP3A4, Drug Metab Lett 2011, 5:183-191

[42] Li AP, Bode C, Sakai Y: A novel in vitro system, the integrated discrete multiple organ cell culture (IdMOC) system, for the evaluation of human drug toxicity: comparative cytotoxicity of tamoxifen towards normal human cells from five major organs and MCF-7 adenocarcinoma breast cancer cells, Chem Biol Interact 2004, 150:129-136

[43] Li AP: In vitro evaluation of human xenobiotic toxicity: scientific concepts and the novel integrated discrete multiple cell co-culture (IdMOC) technology, ALTEX 2008, 25:43-49

[44] Li AP: The use of the Integrated Discrete Multiple Organ Co-culture (IdMOC) system for the evaluation of multiple organ toxicity, Altern Lab Anim 2009, 37:377-385

[45] Morgan RE, Trauner M, van Staden CJ, Lee PH, Ramachandran B, Eschenberg M, Afshari CA, Qualls CW, Jr., Lightfoot-Dunn R, Hamadeh HK: Interference with bile salt export pump function is a susceptibility factor for human liver injury in drug development, Toxicol Sci 2010, 118:485-500

[46] Diao L, Li N, Brayman TG, Hotz KJ, Lai Y: Regulation of MRP2/ABCC2 and BSEP/ABCB11 expression in sandwich cultured human and rat hepatocytes exposed to inflammatory cytokines TNF-{alpha}, IL-6, and IL-1{beta}, J Biol Chem 2010, 285:31185-31192

[47] Maeda K, Sugiyama Y: The use of hepatocytes to investigate drug uptake transporters, Methods Mol Biol 2010, 640:327-353

[48] Rotroff DM, Beam AL, Dix DJ, Farmer A, Freeman KM, Houck KA, Judson RS, LeCluyse EL, Martin MT, Reif DM, Ferguson SS: Xenobiotic-metabolizing enzyme and transporter gene expression in primary cultures of human hepatocytes modulated by ToxCast chemicals, J Toxicol Environ Health B Crit Rev 2010, 13:329-346

[49] Liao M, Raczynski AR, Chen M, Chuang BC, Zhu Q, Shipman R, Morrison J, Lee D, Lee FW, Balani SK, Xia CQ: Inhibition of hepatic organic anion-transporting polypeptide by RNA interference in sandwich-cultured human hepatocytes: an in vitro model to assess transporter-mediated drug-drug interactions, Drug Metab Dispos 2010, 38:1612-1622

[50] Badolo L, Rasmussen LM, Hansen HR, Sveigaard C: Screening of OATP1B1/3 and OCT1 inhibitors in cryopreserved hepatocytes in suspension, Eur J Pharm Sci 2010, 40:282-288

8

The Use of *In Vitro* 3D Cell Models in Drug Development for Respiratory Diseases

Song Huang, Ludovic Wiszniewski and Samuel Constant
Epithelix Sàrl
Switzerland

1. Introduction

In a certain way, drug developers are like the blind men in the well-known tale of "THE BLIND MEN AND THE ELEPHANT", who believe the elephant to be like a water spout, a fan a pillar and a throne since they can only feel a different part but only one part of the elephant's body such as trunk, ear, leg, back. Impossible to test a drug lead on human beings, drug developers also are obliged to forge a whole picture of the "elephant" – how a drug candidate would behave in a whole human body, by using information from the "parts" - models. The task of the drug developers are far more complex and challenging than the blind men, instead of touching only the surface, they have to go deep into the human bodies: organs, tissues, cells, genes, proteins, lipids, hormones ... Furthermore, a living human being is a dynamic and interacting system, in a certain sense, the situation of the drug developers are even worse than the blind men: the blind men touch and feel a real elephant, the information that they get is true; a drug developer, most of the time, works on models, animal models or *in vitro* cell models, which are far from representing a human beings as a whole. As consequences, the information that one gets sometimes could be misleading. For drug developers, the misleading information could have serious consequences in terms of costs and human lives.

This blind men's approach may explain why a drug candidate, even though successfully passed pre-clinical stages, eventually failed at clinical trials. The failure of Torcetrapib, a drug developed by Pfizer, gives an example of just how difficult to develop a drug. Torcetrapib, designed to prevent heart attacks and strokes, is a cholesteryl-ester transfer protein (CETP) inhibitor. Genetic studies of the Japanese populations revealed that people with a deficiency of CETP presented a favorable lipid profile compared with unaffected family members: namely more High Density Lipoproteins (HDL, good) and less Low Density Lipoproteins (LDL, bad) (Inazu et al., 1990; Koizumi et al., 1991). CETP naturally became a target of drug development. Preclinical studies of Torcetrapib on different animal models (mice, rabbits, etc) didn't reveal any severe side effects (Tall et al., 2007). But, medication of Torcetrapib on human beings caused severe hypertension and an increased mortality; apparently there was no obvious beneficial effects on coronary heart disease. The development of Torcetrapib was halted at 2006.

This example illustrates another difficulty in drug development: the genetic heterogeneity of the human populations. The knowledge obtained from one group of people may not be applicable to another group of people. Quite often, this truth has been neglected.

Furthermore, human body is a complex dynamic system, with interconnected networks, equilibrium, feedback, compensation, redundancy, etc..., the cause-effect relationship between the target and the patho-physiological condition is not linear. In the example of CETP, people with the genetic deficiency of CETP, despite of having a favorable lipid profile, also suffer from coronary heart disease (Hirano et al., 1995).

Unfortunately, Torcetrapib is not an exception. According to a statistics, the failure rate at Phase III clinical trials is estimated to be 50% and only 12% of compounds entering into the human phase testing will eventually makes to the market place (Chuang & Stein, 2004).

However, despite of these difficulties, efficient and safe drugs have been successfully developed. The huge increase of the life-span of human populations is the testimony of this success.

The question now is how to improve the success rate of the drug development? In light of the above discussions, we could give a generally recommendations:

1. If possible, use models as close as possible to human patho-physiology and disease conditions.
2. Take into account of the genetic heterogeneity whenever possible during the preclinical studies.
3. Simulate as realistically as possible the dynamic and complex nature of biological responses.

The recent development of 3D human tissue models and the *in silico* models are some attempts to get closer to the human "reality". In this article, authors try to give an overview of the different models for studying the respiratory diseases and for drug development. First of all, in order to develop efficient and safe drugs, it is crucial to understand the nature and the underlying cellular and molecular mechanisms of the pathogenesis of the disease that one would like to treat. In the following sections, we will describe several major respiratory diseases.

2. Respiratory diseases

Respiratory disease is a medical term that encompasses pathological conditions affecting the normal function of the respiratory systems, making the gas exchange impossible. Anatomically, the respiratory system is composed of upper respiratory tract, trachea, bronchi, bronchioles, alveoli, pleura and pleural cavity, and the nerves and muscles of breathing. During the breathing, the respiratory system constantly expose to external insults such as bacteria, virus, particles, gas, etc... making the respiratory system highly vulnerable to various diseases. Indeed, according to the WHO World Health Report 2000, the top five respiratory diseases account for 17.4% of all deaths and 13.3% of all Disability-Adjusted Life Years (DALYs). Lower respiratory tract infections, chronic obstructive pulmonary disease (COPD), tuberculosis and lung cancer are each among the leading 10 causes of death worldwide. There are urgent and unmet needs of better treatments for respiratory diseases.

Respiratory diseases could be classified in various ways. In this article, we will classify them by the cause (etiology) of the disease. As such, the respiratory diseases can be divided into the following categories:

* Inflammatory lung disease
* Obstructive lung diseases
* Respiratory tract infections
* Respiratory tumors

- Pleural cavity diseases
- Pulmonary vascular diseases

We are going to limit our scope to the respiratory tract infections and inflammatory lung diseases. However, it is necessary to point out that one disease may be classified in several categories. For example, asthma is caused by airway inflammation; the consequence is the airway obstruction. Viral infection may also contribute to asthma exacerbation. The interplay of multi-factorial risks makes the drug development even more challenging.

2.1 Respiratory tract infections

Over 200 different viruses have been isolated in patients with respiratory tract infections. The most common virus is the rhinovirus. Other viruses include the coronavirus, parainfluenza virus, adenovirus, enterovirus, and respiratory syncytial virus (RSV) (Mäkelä et al., 1998). Up to 15% of acute pharyngitis cases may be caused by bacteria, commonly Group A streptococcus in Streptococcal pharyngitis ("Strep Throat") (Bisno, 2001). Influenza (the flu) is a more severe systemic illness which typically involves the upper respiratory tract.

During evolution, the viruses as well as bacteria co-evolve and adapt to their host, acquiring so-called tropism, namely the specificity of a given virus or bacterium for a cell type, tissue or species. The well known example is the influenza viruses. Certain strains of influenza A viruses such as H5N1 infect specifically one species: avian, pig, or human, etc... Thanks to this species barrier, the deadly avian H5N1 has not been able to cause "pandemics" within human populations.

Even though there are several determinants of the viral tropism, the main molecular basis of the viral tropism is the specific cell surface receptor(s) for viral entry. A typical and well-studied example is the receptors for influenza viruses (Fig.1. and Fig.2.).

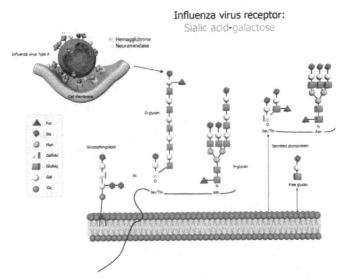

Fig. 1. Schematic representation of the interaction of Influenza virus and its receptors.On the apical surface of the airway epithelial cells, most of the membrane proteins are glycosylated on serine (O-glycan) or asparagine (N-glycan). The glycans are often have a sialic acid (sia) tail linked to galactose (gal), which serves as receptor for Influenza A viruses such as H1N1.

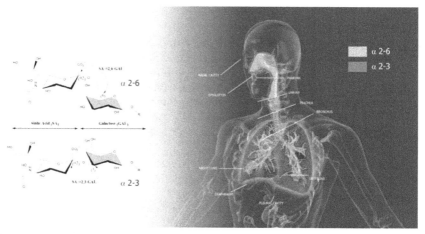

Fig. 2. Two types of linkages which plays an important role in viral tropism. Avian Influenza A viruses prefer α2-3 linkage, human Influenza A viruses, α2-6, porcine Influenza A viruses are adapted to both α2-3 and α2-6. In the human lung, there exists a particular distribution pattern of these two linkages: α2-6 linkage is present mainly on the airway epithelial surface lining the respiratory tracts, from the nose down to the bronchioles. In contrast, α2-3 linkage is located in the alveolar cavity mainly on the type-II cells.

The receptor of influenza A virus is glycosylated-proteins with a terminal sialic acid linked to galactose. There exist two main types of linkages: SA-α2-3-Gal and SA-α2-6-Gal. It has been shown that the avian Influenza A viruses prefer α2-3 linkage, human Influenza A viruses, α2-6, porcine Influenza A viruses are adapted to both α2-3 and α2-6.

What is interesting is the distribution of these two types of linkage in human airway epithelial cells. Using lectin probes specific for each type of linkages, the distribution of these two types of linkages has been studied in the human lungs (Shinya et al., 2006; Van Riel et al., 2006). It has been demonstrated that epithelial cells in the paranasal sinuses, the pharynx, the trachea, the bronchi as well as in the terminal and respiratory bronchioles, mainly express SA-α2-6-Gal. In contrast, SA-α2-3-Gal was found on non-ciliated cuboidal bronchiolar cells at the junction between the respiratory bronchiole and alveolus, and a substantial number of cells lining the alveolar wall also expressed this molecule. Moreover, the SA-α2-3-Gal-positive alveolar cells also reacted to an antibody against surfactant protein A; this suggests that they were alveolar type-II cells (which express surfactant proteinA) (Shinya et al., 2006; Van Riel et al., 2006).

Using similar approach, Varki and Varki confirmed these results. Moreover, they discovered that this distribution pattern seems to be unique of human lungs, it is even absent in the lung of great apes (Varki & Varki 2009).

Since most of the bacteria infect the human respiratory tracts without entering into the cells, the tropism of bacteria is less evident. But, in certain physiological as well as pathological conditions, bacteria preferentially infect certain species or tissues. As example, in patients suffering from cystic fibrosis (the pathology will be discussed below), the respiratory tracts of the patients are chronically colonized by *P. aeruginosa* which can rarely be eradicated. This chronic infection provokes lung inflammation and lung injury, leading to respiratory failure and death (Kerem et al., 1990). The reason of this persistent infection by *P. aeruginosa* is still not clear. But it is reasonable to assume that the respiratory tracts of the CF patients provide a niche particularly favorable to *P. aeruginosa*.

So, given these particular and unique pathogen and host relationship, it is preferable to use human models for drug development for treating viral and bacterial infections of the human respiratory tracts.

2.2 Inflammatory lung diseases

Another category of respiratory diseases is the inflammatory lung diseases such as asthma, cystic fibrosis, emphysema, chronic obstructive pulmonary, characterized by a high neutrophil count. The mechanisms of immune responses in cystic fibrosis, asthma, COPD diseases have been extensively documented. The common feature of these inflammatory airway diseases is the involvement of the respiratory airway epithelia.

Cystic fibrosis (CF) is an autosomal recessive, a multisystem disorder, characterized primarily by defective electrolyte transport in **epithelial cells** and abnormally viscid mucus secretions from glands and mucus epithelia. The impairment of the mucociliary clearance leads to chronic infection and inflammation, ultimately causing cystic bronchiectasis, severe airflow obstruction and death (Boucher, 2004, 2007) (Figure 3).

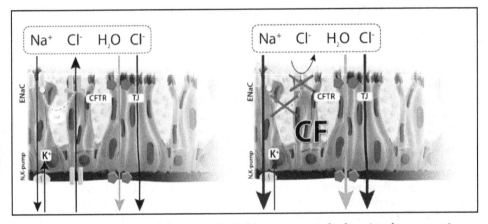

Fig. 3. Schema depicts normal airway epithelial ion transport, dysfunctional transport in CF.Normal airway epithelia (left): CFTR functions as a Cl- and it also regulates Na+ absorption (it inhibits ENaC). The quantity of NaCl on airway surface is optimally regulated to osmotically hydrate the periciliary and mucus layers allowing efficient mucus clearance. CF airway epithelia (right): In the absence of the CFTR protein in the apical membrane consequent to common CF mutations, such as ΔF508 CFTR, the CF epithelium can exhibit unrestrained Na+ absorption and a failure to secrete Cl-. These combined defects reduce the quantity of NaCl on CF airway surfaces, maintain less water osmotically on CF airway surfaces and, hence, lead to depletion of water in the periciliary liquid layer (PCL) and collapse of a thickened mucus layer onto the epithelial surface.

Asthma is an inflammatory disease characterized by allergic reaction to allergens and chemicals. The hallmark of asthma diseases is the antigen-specific IgE production. Even though the effector cells in asthma pathogenesis are immune cells like dendritic cells, helper

T cells (usually CD4+ cells), eosinophils, neutrophils, etc... the airway epithelia play an important role in the induction phase of asthma. Indeed, recent advances suggest that a cytokine named Thymic Stromal Lymphopoietin (TSLP) might play a key role in biasing the Th0 cells to Th2 differentiation pathway (Rochman et al., 2008; Ziegler et al., 2006; Esnault et al., 2008; Shi et al., 2008). What is more, TSLPR-knock-out mice failed to develop lung inflammation upon ovalbumin challenge (Al-Shami et al., 2005). Conversely, the over-expression of TSLP in mice induces spontaneous airway inflammation and atopic dermatis (Zhou et al., 2005; Yoo et al., 2005), suggesting TSLP is an important factor necessary and sufficient for the initiation of allergic airway inflammation. The implication of TSLP in Th2 response is further confirmed by studies of other allergic diseases such as the skin atopic dermatis (Zhou et al., 2005) and intestinal immune homeostasis (Zaph et al., 2007). Interestingly, expression of TSLP is elevated in the bronchial biopsies from the asthmatic patients compared to that of healthy donors (Ying et al., 2005).

Chronic Obstructive Pulmonary Disease (COPD) is now the fifth leading cause of death worldwide (Pauwels & Rabe, 2004) and it will become, as predicted by the World Health Organization (WHO), the third leading cause of death worldwide by 2030 (www.who.int/respiratory/copd/en/index.html). Even though airborne pollutants such as smoke from the burning fuel or coals can cause COPD, the main inducing factor is the cigarette smoke. COPD is a complex syndrome comprised of airway inflammation, mucociliary dysfunction and consequent airway structural destruction. This process is considered non-reversible.

Upon the irritant challenge, the airway epithelial cells synthesize and release pro-inflammatory cytokines and chemokines such as IL-8, MIP-3α, which in turn recruit neutrophils, CD8+ T-lymphocytes, B-Cells, macrophages and dendritic cells to the lumen of the airways. The matrix-metalloproteinases (MMP-6, MMP-9), among other mediators, cause airway injury and remodeling, eventually leading to airway obstruction.

3. The Airway epithelium: Central to the pathogenesis of respiratory diseases

From the above descriptions, it is clear that the airway epithelial cells occupy a central position in the pathogenesis of most respiratory diseases, ranging from infectious diseases, genetic diseases, to most inflammatory diseases. Indeed, it has been long recognized that the airway epithelium is more than just a barrier: it synthesizes and releases a large panel of chemokines, cytokines, lipids, growth factors, proteases, protease inhibitors, for example, IL-8, Il-6, IL-17F, TGFs (Folkerts et al., 1998; Laberge et al., 2004; Suzuki et al., 2007). And the expression of these cytokines and chemokines are induced and modulated by various external insults like viral and bacterial infections, cigarette smokes (Nakamura et al., 2008) and are associated with disease conditions like CF, asthma, and COPD (Fig. 4).

This paradigm provides a theoretic framework for developing more relevant *in vitro* cells models of allergic asthma and COPD, especially the *in vitro* 3D cell models of the human airway epithelium.

4. The experimental models

A survey of the existing models of respiratory diseases may be useful for the readers. Knowing the strengths and limitations of each model will help drug developers to choose the more appropriate tools for their work.

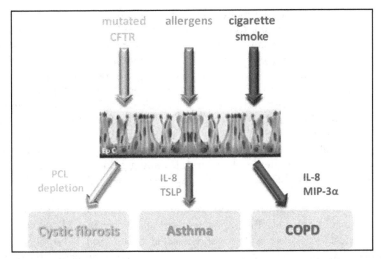

Fig. 4. The Airway epithelium - central to the pathogenesis of respiratory diseases. In addition to its barrier functions, the airway epithelium is also an immune-modulator involved in most of the respiratory diseases.

4.1 Animal models

Animal models are widely used for studying the respiratory diseases and for drug development. Due to the economical and technical reasons, the small rodents like mice and rats are the most popular and widely used animal models. Besides, chicken eggs, rabbits, guinea pig, cats, dogs, sheep, monkeys are also routinely used (Epstein, 2004).

For example, embryonated chicken eggs have been extensively used for growing the influenza viruses and for vaccine production (Potkin & Potkin, 2006; Artenstein, 2009). However, since the dominant linkage in the embryonated chicken eggs is α2-3, some of the field strains grow poorly or not at all in chicken eggs. Furthermore, High mutation rates of RNA viruses like Influenza A allow the generation of viral escape mutants, rendering vaccines and drugs directed against virus encoded targets potentially ineffective (Neumann et al., 2009). A new strategy is to temporarily disable the host cellular factors necessary for viral replication, thus reduce the risk of selecting for resistant viral mutants. Using genome-wide RNAi screen approach, Karlas et al. have identified hundreds of human host factors crucial for influenza A virus (H5N1) replication in A459 cells (Karlas et al., 2010). However, Due to the genetic drift of A549, a cancerous alveolar cell line, it is necessary to confirm these results in primary human pneumocytes. As discussed above, the major concern about pandemic threat of avian influenza A is the possibility of avian flu virus to acquire the ability to infect the upper human airway tracts which are rich in α2-6 linkage.

As animal models, mice and rats are routinely used for studying respiratory diseases. Besides the economical considerations, the biggest advantage of rodent models is the possibility to modify genetically the animals. Indeed, transgenic mice with knock-out CFTR or with delta-F508 mutations have been created (Colledge et al., 1992; Snouwaert et al., 1992; Ratcliff et al., 1993; O'Neal et al., 1993; Hasty et al., 1995). Unfortunately, these transgenic mice don't present lung problems as found in cystic fibrosis patients, highlighting once again the molecular, cellular and physiological differences between animals and human.

As for asthma and COPD animal models, since the rodents don't naturally develop these human diseases, allergic asthma or COPD has to be induced artificially by immunizing and challenging the respiratory tracts with antigen/allergen or proteases/cigarette smokes (for reviews: Epstein, 2008; Churg et al., 2008). Even though some asthmatic symptoms like eosinophil infiltration, mucus hypersecretion, airway hyper responsiveness, and elevated IgE production, can be observed, the lung inflammation is often transient rather than chronic as in human being. Similarly, due to the considerable differences of lung anatomy and susceptibility to injurious agents among species (Bracke et al., 2007), none of the animal COPD models reproduces the exact changes seen in humans (Churg et al., 2008).

Occasionally, naturally occurring animal disease models could also be found and used. For example, Ascaris suum-allergic sheep and flea-allergic dog have been discovered and used for studying asthma diseases and for drug development (Singh et al., 2002; Tang et al., 2003).

One way to get closer to human disease conditions, so-called humanized animal models have also been made to explore the pathogenesis of allergic asthma: the human peripheral blood mononuclear cells were isolated and injected into T and B lymphocyte deficient severe combined immunodeficiency (SCID) mice, creating a human-SCID mouse. Even though it is an innovative approach, due to the complexity of the human immune systems, it is not possible to humanize all the immune cells of the SCID mouse.

In short, animal models, even though useful, indispensable and informative, don't give the true picture of the human respiratory diseases. Sometimes, it is even misleading. Furthermore, none of these animal models can reflect the human genetic heterogeneity which is key for developing safe and efficient drugs.

4.2 Human respiratory disease models
There are several categories of human disease models:
- Cell lines
- Primary cells
- 3D cell models
- Cell co-cultures
- Explants
- *In silico* models

Until now, the most popular human models are cell lines derived from various human tissues.

4.2.1 Epithelial cell lines
The airway epithelia constitute the first line of defense against the external insults. It has a pseudo-layer structure consisted of three main types of cells: ciliated epithelial cells, mucus cells and basal cells. The mucus cells synthesize and secret mucin-rich mucus which trap most of the inhaled particles, virus and bacteria, the later are eliminated from the body by muco-cilliary clearance via the cilia-beating. All the three cell types contribute to the pathogenesis of respiratory diseases, for example, inflammatory reaction, mucus hypersecretion, airway remodeling (Epstein, 2004; Verstraelen et al., 2008).

As airway epithelial cell lines, the most frequently used ones are A549, BEAS-2B, Calu3, 16HBE14o-, etc... The characteristics and uses of these cell lines have been nicely reviewed by Verstraelen et al., 2008.

A549

Origin: This line was initiated in 1972 by D.J. Giard, et al. (Giard, 1972) through explant culture of lung carcinomatous tissue from a 58-year-old Caucasian male. As type II pulmonary epithelial cells (alveolar pneumocyte), it synthesizes lecithin with a high percentage of disaturated fatty acids (surfactants). It is oncogenic when tested in nude mice. *Applications*: The cells can be used to screen chemical and biological agents for ability to induce or affect differentiation and/or carcinogenesis. Mechanistic studies, pathway-mapping and target-finding, or ranking of the toxicity potency of chemicals.

BEAS-2B

Origin: BEAS-2B cells were isolated from normal human bronchial epithelium obtained from autopsy of non-cancerous individuals. The cells were infected and immortalized with an adenovirus 12-SV40 virus hybrid Ad12SV40 and cloned. These cells retain the ability to undergo squamous differentiation in response to serum, and stained positively for keratins and SV40 T antigen.
Applications: The cells can be used to test the toxicity of chemicals and biological agents relevant to upper airway epithelia. Suitable for mechanistic studies, pathway-mapping and target-finding.

Calu-3

Unlike most immortal cells, Calu-3 cells form sheets of cells that are welded to each other by tight junctions. These sheets form a fully functional epithelium that can transport large quantities of ions and fluid. In addition, Calu-3 cells have the highest level of natural CFTR expression of any known immortalized cell, even higher than some intestinal cell lines that once held the record. Thus, this cell line is suitable to study cystic fibrosis and drug discovery (Haws et al., 1994).

4.2.2 Immune cells (Effector cells)

Dendritic cells: Although both the skin and lung airway mucosa possess resident dendritic cells, the majority of studies conducted to date have utilized human peripheral blood mononuclear cell-derived dendritic cells (PBMC-DC) due to their relative ease of extraction and the ability to obtain larger quantities of cells (Casati et al., 2005). Several protocols have been established to generate human DC *in vitro*. Starting with blood or bone marrow-derived CD34+ hematopoietic progenitor cells (HPC), DC can be generated under various culture conditions with a cocktail of specific cytokines. Despite of the progress made in the field, it is still difficult to obtain sufficient amount of primary DC cell for basic or clinic research. Therefore, the use of cell lines such as THP-1, KG-1, especially the MUTZ-3, proves to be invaluable (Santegoets et al., 2008).

Mast cells, neutrophils, eosinophils, , basophils, are considered as effector cells which are involved in early and late phases of asthma by releasing a plethora of inflammatory mediators. Their roles in broncho-constriction, mucus secretion, and airway remodeling have clearly defined. Many therapeutics are targeting these effector cells and associated key molecules (Casale et al., 2008). These cells can be isolated from the blood or cord blood and cultured *in vitro*. Their behaviors such as migration, free radical production, viability and apoptosis, can be assessed after stimulation by allergen and cytokines (Frieri et al., 2003; Tang et al., 2003; Nilsson et al., 2004).

4.2.3 The drawbacks of cell lines

1. These cells have been transformed by oncogenes one way or other, thus certain signal transduction networks have been deregulated.
2. Genetic aberrations such as chromosomes loss, chromosomes translation, mutations, etc…
3. These cell lines cannot give rise to fully differentiated phenotypes of the original tissues such as cilia formation, mucus secretion, epithelium repair and remodeling.
4. Under the monolayer culture conditions, the cells behave totally different as they do in vivo situations. These differences have been illustrated by comparing the responses of the same cancer cells to drugs (Bissell et al., 2006; Yamada et al., 2006; Griffith & Schartz, 2006).

4.2.4 Fully differentiated 3D human airway epithelial models

To overcome these shortcomings of the cell lines, different techniques have been developed to make 3 dimensional (3D) cultures, by providing a micro-environment or architecture closer to *in vivo* situations. Among these techniques, cellular matrix scaffold, hang-drop culture, perfusion culture chambers, air-liquid interface cultures, etc…

However, in order to simulate the *in vivo* lung conditions, the ALI cultures seem to be more appropriate: the basal-lateral side of the epithelia is immerged in the culture medium and the apical side is exposed to humidified air with 5% CO_2. Furthermore, with the Costar PET Transwell inserts, it is very practical and convenient to use. It is suitable for most of the applications, such as imaging, immune-cytochemistry, toxicity tests, electrophysiological studies (Ussing chamber measurement), assessment of drug permeation and drug formulations, etc…

4.2.4.1 MucilAir

It is a fully differentiated and ready-to-use 3D model of human airway epithelium, constituted with primary human epithelial cells freshly isolated from the nasal or bronchial biopsies. It is commercially available and ready-to-use (Epithelix, www.epithelix.com). MucilAir (Fig. 5.), is not only morphologically and functionally differentiated, but also can also be maintained in a homeostatic state for a long period of time. Using cells from diseased donors, different versions of MucilAir can be made such as asthmatic, allergic, COPD, CF, etc…

4.2.4.2 Applications of MucilAir in drug development

Due to its fully differentiated nature, MucilAir can be used for studying various respiratory diseases. In the following paragraphs, we will give some examples about the applications of MucilAir in drug development.

4.2.4.2.1 Viral infections

MucilAir has been successfully used for studying Pandemic H1N1 2009 influenza virus (Brookes et al., 2010). It is also suitable for other respiratory viruses like Respiratory syncytial virus (RSV) and Human Rhinovirus (HRV) (Fig. 6.). The results are highly reproducible.

4.2.4.2.2 Electro-physiology of the airway epithelia (Ussing chamber measurements)

One of the characteristics of the airway epithelia is the active ion transport which is essential for regulating and maintaining the ion composition and height of the pericilliary liquid layer. The ion channel activities of the airway epithelia can be monitored in a modified Ussing Chamber. In the following figure, the short circuit current mediated by CFTR is absent when stimulated with Isoproterenol which increases the intra-cellular cyclic AMP (see above discussion on CF pathology). Typical recording is shown in Fig. 7.. Related to electrophysiology is the muco-ciliary clearance. It is convenient to use MucilAir for evaluating the drug effects on cilia beating and muco-ciliary clearance.

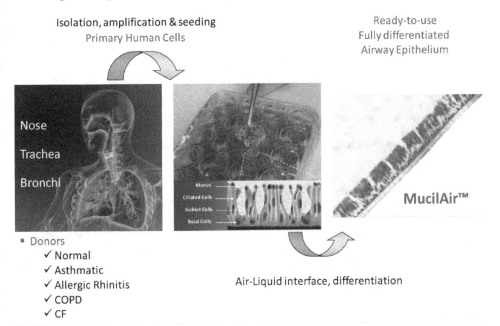

Fig. 5. MucilAir, a fully differentiated 3D in vitro cell model of the human airway epithelia Epithelial cells were freshly isolated from the biopsies (nose, trachea, and bronchi), then seeded onto a semi-porous membrane (Costar Transwell, pore size 0.4 μm). After about 45 days of culture at air-liquid interface, the epithelia were fully differentiated, both morphologically and functionally. Depending on the pathology of the donors, different versions of MucilAir could be made.

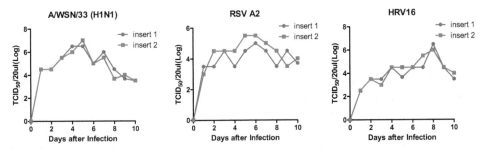

Fig. 6. MucilAir was infected apically: A/WSN/33, H1N1 influenza, 1MOI; RSV A2, 0.1MOI; HRV16, 1MOI. The virions were collected by washing the apical surface with 500 μl culture medium. The titre of the viruses was measured by ELISA.

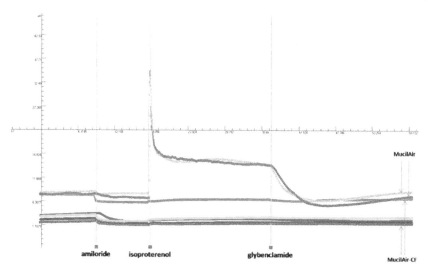

Fig. 7. Measurement of the short-circuit current in modified Ussing chambers. The reconstituted epithelia are placed in modified Ussing chambers and the short-circuit currents are measured after the addition of various blockers and activators of the ionic channels. Addition of Amiloride (blocker of the sodium channels) reduced the current. The addition of Isoproterenol increased the current in normal MucilAir, but in MucilAir-CF. The addition of glybenclamide (an inhibitor of CFTR channel) completely inhibited the currents mediated by CFTR in normal MucilAir.

4.2.4.2.3 Mucociliary clearance analysis

The muco-ciliary clearance is the principal defense mechanism of the respiratory systems. The impairment of this function is the major cause of chronic infection and inflammation, as exemplified in cystic fibrosis disease. For experimental reasons, direct measurements of mucus velocity in human lungs are presently available only for the trachea, with values ranged from 4-6 mm/min. (Hofmann et al., 2002). The only reported value of the mucus velocity in the main bronchi is about 2.4 mm/min (Foster et al., 1982). Interestingly, the same value has been obtained by using an in vitro culture model of the bronchial airway epithelial cells (Masui et al., 1998). However, the velocity of muco-ciliary clearance varies considerable depending on individuals, anatomical location, and disease conditions, etc... Indeed, the values that we obtained from the nasal epithelia are slightly inferior to that of bronchial ones, about 1.8 mm/min (Fig. 8.). Due to the simplicity of *in vitro* methods, it is possible to access the drug effects on muco-ciliary clearance in various disease settings.

4.2.4.2.4 Multi-endpoint test strategy

In addition to its applications in viral infection and cystic fibrosis, MucilAir can also be used for testing the toxicity and efficacy of the drugs candidates. To this end, a multi-endpoint strategy is used (Fig. 9.). The drug candidates can be applied on the apical surface as liquids, solids, gaz, smoke and nanoparticles. The effects of drugs can be monitored by several endpoints: such as the trans-epithelial electric resistance (TEER), cell viability tests (Resazurin, LDH), cilia beating frequency monitoring, muco-ciliary clearance, mucus secretion, release of cytokines/chemokines.

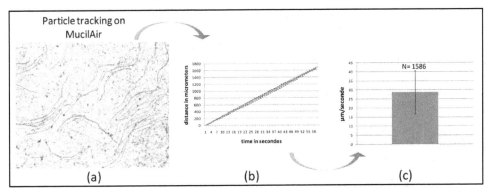

Fig. 8. Due to its fully differentiated nature, muco-ciliary clearance can be easily studied in vitro on MucilAir. Briefly, the mucociliary clearance is monitored using a fully automated setup dedicated to video-microscopy. Microbeads of 5 microns are seeded onto the apical surface of MucilAir-normal or MucilAir-CF cultures. Then, pictures are taken every second during 1 minute in order to reconstitute movies showing the movement of the small particles. The particle movement is then tracked using dedicated software for calculating velocities of beads' movement.

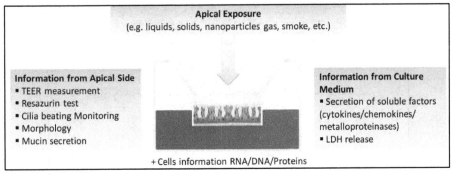

Fig. 9. Multiple end points testing strategy for toxicity testing using MucilAir

4.2.4.2.5 Dextran application

One of the problems that drug developers frequently encounter is the solubility of the compounds: not all the chemicals are soluble or stable in solutions. It is also difficult to test powders or nanoparticles. In order to solve this problem, a procedure which allows testing all kinds of solid substances was developed (PCT/IB2010/053956). The idea is to use inert and neutral substances as carrier. Dextran was successfully used as carrier to deliver the insoluble chemical compounds and nanoparticles onto the apical surfaces of MucilAir. Dextran is a bacterial byproduct; the dextran macromolecule consists of glycan groups linked end to end. It didn't show any harmful effect on MucilAir. The following figure describes the procedure and application of the dextran tablets (Fig. 10.).

4.2.4.2.6 Simulation of chronic airway inflammation

Airway epithelium is more than just a barrier; it is also an immune-modulator. Upon external stimulations, it synthesizes and releases a large panel of chemokines, cytokines, lipids, growth factors, proteases, protease inhibitors. In the following figure (Fig. 11.), the epithelia were repetitively stimulated by Cytomix (TNF-α/LPS). It is remarkable that the airway epithelial cells could recover after repetitive challenge of Cytomix, a relatively physiological stimulus. It was not the cases with some chemical compounds (data not shown).

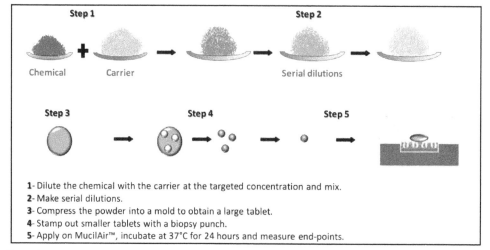

1- Dilute the chemical with the carrier at the targeted concentration and mix.
2- Make serial dilutions.
3- Compress the powder into a mold to obtain a large tablet.
4- Stamp out smaller tablets with a biopsy punch.
5- Apply on MucilAir™, incubate at 37°C for 24 hours and measure end-points.

Fig. 10. Preparation and application of the Dextran Tablets

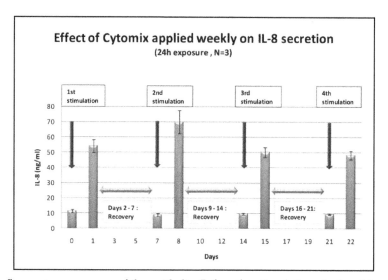

Fig. 11. Inflammatory response of the epithelia. Before the stimulation, the basal level of IL-8 was about 10 ng/ml. After 24 hours of stimulation with pro-inflammatory mediators (Cytomix = TNF-α + LPS), the amount of IL-8 released was increased five-fold. Upon removal of the stimulus, the amount of IL-8 returned to basal level as day 0. The epithelia could respond to the stimulus in a physiological manner again and again.

4.2.4.2.7 Repeated dose and long term toxicity testing using MucilAir

Quite often, it is necessary to perform repeated dose and Long term toxicity/efficacy test of drug candidates. Up to now, this kind of experiments can be performed only on animals. In the following graph, we provide a proof-of-concept for repeated dose tests using an *in vitro* cell model. It is a transposition of the OECD412 guideline for 28 day test on rodents. The TEER was used as endpoint, which is an indicator of the epithelial integrity (Fig. 12.). This is a very sensitive endpoint. The "No Observed Adverse Effect Level"(NOAEL) can be determined (around 10 mM).

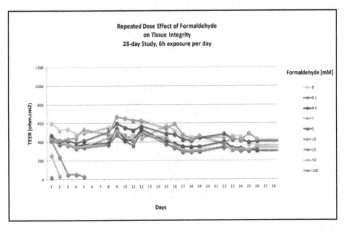

Fig. 12. Repeated dose tests of formaldehyde on MucilAir (28 days repeated dose exposure study). 6 hours per day exposure on MucilAir to Formaldehyde for a period of 28 days. Every day, tissue Integrity (TEER) were measured (N=3) then epithelia were reused for the next exposure.

4.2.4.2.8 Drug permeation

In recent decades, the nasal mucosa has become an established administration site for systemic as well as local drug delivery (Ugwoke et al., 2005). For developing novel drugs intended for this route, reliable methods are needed for assessing the rate and extent of absorption across the nasal epithelium. Desired methods should enable studies of enhancer effects and toxicology. By transposing the Caco-2 protocol (Hubatsch et al., 2007) to MucilAir™, trans-epithelial permeability of drug candidates or xenobiotics can be assessed on MucilAir™. Since epithelium is grown on separable inserts, kinetic studies are facilitated (Fig. 13.). The results obtained are very similar using different batches of MucilAir™ derived from different donors. Apical to basolateral and basolateral to apical permeability studies on height reference compound were performed (Table 1).

4.2.4.2.9 The problem of variability

One of the concerns of using the primary human cells is the variability from donor to donor: researchers don't like variability! Indeed, one of the gold standards of scientific analysis is the reproducibility. If one performs an experiment with a standard operating protocol, one should get the same results. We agree with this principle. But, the genetic heterogeneity of the human population is a reality that drug developers have to face sooner or later: Exposed to the same allergens, only a small percent of people develop asthma. Not all the smokers suffer from COPD. This reality has to be taken into account whenever possible, and as early as possible. Thus, in our opinion, the donor-dependent variation is not a problem; on the contrary, it could be a solution for reducing failure rate at later stages. Using a large collection of frozen primary airway epithelial cells, it is possible to address the issue of the genetic heterogeneity of the human populations. With tools like genomics, proteomics, bio-informatics, etc, it would be possible to pin down cellular and molecular mechanisms underlying the donor to donor variability.

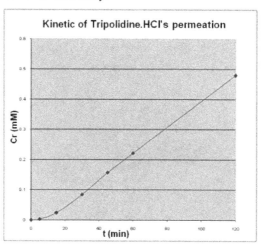

Fig. 13. Time course of the rate of permeability of Tripolidine.HCl from the apical to basolateral side (N=3).

Molecules	Papp (cm/s) A→B	Papp (cm/s) B→A	Asymmetry Ratio
Salicilic Acid	7.7×10^{-5}	1.7×10^{-5}	0.2
Nicotine	2.1×10^{-5}	3.3×10^{-5}	1.6
Propranolol. HCl	1.2×10^{-5}	1.6×10^{-5}	1.3
Ibuprofen	1.1×10^{-5}	1.9×10^{-5}	1.7
Tripolidine. HCl	9.7×10^{-6}	1.2×10^{-5}	1.2
Tetracaïne. HCl	8.0×10^{-6}	1.1×10^{-5}	1.3
Dopamine. HCl	3.0×10^{-6}	2.5×10^{-6}	0.8
Atenolol	2.2×10^{-6}	6.7×10^{-6}	3.0

Table 1. Evaluation of transport of 8 reference compounds across MucilAir (N=3)

4.2.5 Immune competent 3D models

Despite the central rule of the airway epithelia, other cellular components are also implicated and necessary for understanding the pathology of respiratory diseases, especially the immune cells.

Co-culture systems: To study the cross-talks between different types of cells, the simplest way is by co-culturing different cells involved *in vitro*. Such experiments have been carried out using established cell lines: for examples, BEAS-2B are co-cultured with human lung fibroblasts (HFL-1 or WISTAR-38) (Lang et al., 1998), human umbilical vein endothelial cells (ECV304) (Mögel et al., 1998), or eosinophils (Wong et al., 2005), and primary human BECs with alveolar macrophages (Ishii et al., 2005). Using 3D cell models like MucilAir™ and freshly isolated immune cells, more reliable and faithful co-culture systems could be developed for studying the inflammatory respiratory diseases like asthma or COPD diseases and for drug development.

Explants: Another way is to use explants. In other words, part of animal or human lung was excised and cultured *in vitro* for a period of days or weeks. The effects of cytokines or chemical compounds on bronco-constriction have been studied (Wohlsen et al., 2003). Using explants models it is possible to assess immunomodulatory effects (Tan et al., 2009) and understand signaling processes involved in tissue hyperresponsiveness related to asthma (Morin et al., 2005). Precision Cut Lung Slides (PCLS) are now used for studying the effects of sensitizers. PCLS mirrors the complex interplay of different cell types in the living organ and allows physiological processes to be mimicked (Henjakovic et al., 2008). The problem with the lung explants is the rapid degradation of the tissue slices. It is also difficult to obtain health, normal tissues.

Lung on a chip: Ideal is to reconstitute the lung on a chip. Some attempts have been made. For example, Ingber's lab designed and constructed a microfluidics system, so-called Lung on a chip that reproduces both the lung's alveolar-capillary interface and the mechanical effects of breathing on that interface—all on a polymer chip about 2 cm long (Huh et al., 2010). Another example is a so-called **Multi-Compartmental Bioreactor** designed on the basis of allometric scaling laws in order to recreate physiological life conditions of four different human cell types (pancreatic, adipocyte, endothelial and hepatic cells), interconnected each other through media flow (Vozzi et al., 2011). Some physiologically relevant results have been obtained by Vozzi and coworkers, suggesting that interactions, mediated by metabolites present in media flow, have a remarkable effect more than the physical interaction and can lead to a restoration of physiological cell life conditions.

By incorporating the immune cells into these microfluidics systems, it is possible to build an immune-competent human *in vitro* lung model for studying the inflammatory respiratory diseases like asthma and COPD.

4.3 *In silico models*: A systems biological approach - virtual cells, virtual organs, and virtual patients

Despite the spectacular successes of molecular biology, some scientists did feel the drawbacks of the "blind men's approach", and they tried to take a more holistic viewpoint to describe the biological systems (von Bertalanffy, 1968; Noble, 2006). Back to 1960, Noble already developed the first computer model of the heart pacemaker (Noble, 1960). From 2000 onward, so-called systems biology has been gaining popularity and importance. The systems biology tries to put the parts - head, ear, trunk, and legs - together to form a whole elephant: namely to achieve a holistic, quantitative, and predictive understanding through mathematical models that enable an iterative cycle between prediction and experiments (Sauer et al., 2007). Based on systemwide component identification and quantification ("omics" data) at the level of mRNA, proteins, and small molecular weight metabolites, Ishii et al. made a "virtual cell" which includes both the constituting components and the functional state of a metabolic network, providing a proof-of-concept for integrating a heterogeneous data set into a coherent whole (Ishii et al., 2007).

With increasing calculation capacity and better software, it is now possible to simulate more realistically the biological processes at all levels: molecular interaction (ligand-receptor), virtual cells, virtual organs, and even virtual patients (Epstein et al., 2004). The *in silico* approach allows to rapidly integrating new data and novel knowledge, and it can get better and better with time. It is reasonable to hope that in the near future, based on systemwide data collection using relevant human 3D cell/tissue models, we could build a virtual lung for studying the respiratory diseases and for new drug development.

5. Conclusion

Each model has its strengths and weaknesses and there is no perfect respiratory disease model. Depending on the goal or on application, one model could be better than another. Since the drugs are to be used by human beings, it is logic to assess the toxicity and efficacy on cells of human origin, especially on 3D human models. Due to its central role in pathogenesis of respiratory diseases, the 3D *in vitro* cell models of the human airway epithelium deserve more attention in the future. We believe that the 3D cell models like MucilAir are highly relevant and valuable for development of new drugs.

6. Acknowledgments

The authors thank Dr. Kazuhiro Ito from Respivert Ltd. (London) for providing the data on viral infections on MucilAir reported in Fig.6. We also thank the "Ligue Suisse Contre la Vivisection" and the "Fondation E. Naëf pour la recherche *in vitro*" (Geneva) for their continuous support.

7. References

Al-Shami, A. et al. (2005) A role for TSLP in the development of inflammation in an asthma model. *J. Exp. Med.* 202, 829–839

Anderson, M.P., Berger, H.A., Rich, D.P., Gregory, R.J., Smith, A.E. and Welsh, M.J. (1991) Nucleoside triphosphates are required to open the CFTR chloride channel. *Cell*, 67, 775–784.

Artenstein, A.W (2009) "Influenza" In: Vaccines: A Biography Andrew W. Artenstein, ed. pp. 191-205.

Bear, C.E.; Li, C.; Kartner, N.; Bridges, R.J.; Jensen, T.J.; Ramjeesingh, M. and Riordan, J.R. (1992) Purification and functional reconstitution of the cystic fibrosis transmembrane conductance regulator (CFTR). *Cell*, 68, 809–818.

Bisno, A.L. (2001) Acute pharyngitis. *N Engl J Med*: 344:205

Bissell M.J. and LaBarge M.A. (2005) Context, tissue plasticity, and cancer: Are tumor stem cells also regulated by the microenvironment? *Cancer Cell* 7: 17–23

Bracke K.R.; D'hulst A.I.; Maes T; Demedts I.K.; Moerloose K.B.; Kuziel W.A.; Joos G.F.; Brusselle G.G. (2007). Cigarette smoke-induced pulmonary inflammation, but not airway remodelling, is attenuated in chemokine receptor 5-deficient mice. *Clin Exp Allergy* 37: 1467–1479

Casale, T.B. and Stokes, J.R. (2008) Immunomodulators for allergic respiratory disorders. *J Allergy Clin Immunol* 121 (2), 288–296; quiz 297–288

Cheng, S.H.; Rich, D.P.; Marshall, J.; Gregory, R.J.; Welsh, M.J. and Smith, A.E. (1991) Phosphorylation of the R domain by cAMPdependent protein kinase regulates the CFTR chloride channel. *Cell*, 66, 1027–1036

Cheung, M. and Akabas, M.H. (1996) Identification of cystic fibrosis transmembrane conductance regulator channel-lining residues in and flanking the M6 membrane-spanning segment. *Biophys. J.*, 70, 2688–2695

Chuang-Stein, C. (2004). "Seize the opportunities." *Pharmaceutical Statistics.* 3, 157–159

Colledge, W.H.; Ratcliff, R.; Foster, D.; Williamson, R. and Evans, M.J. (1992) Cystic fibrosis mouse with intestinal obstruction. *Lancet*, 340: 680

Esnault, S. et al. (2008) Thymic stromal lymphopoietin (TSLP) as a bridge between infection and atopy. *Int. J. Clin. Exp. Pathol.* 1, 325–330

Epstein, M.M. (2004) Do mouse models of allergic asthma mimic clinical disease? *Int Arch Allergy Immunol* 133 (1), 84-100

Folkerts, G. and Nijkamp, F.P. (1998) Airway epithelium: more than just a barrier! *Trends Pharmacol. Sci.* 19, 334–341

Foster, W. M.; Langenback, E. G. and Bergofsky, E. H. (1982). Lung mucociliary function in man: Interdependence of bronchial and tracheal mucus transport velocities with lung clearance in bronchial asthma and healthy subjects. *Ann. Occup. Hyg.* 26, 227–244.

Friend, S.L. et al. (1994) A thymic stromal cell line supports *in vitro* development of surface IgM+ B cells and produces a novel growth factor affecting B and T lineage cells. *Exp. Hematol.* 22, 321–328

Frieri, M. et al. (2003) Montelukast inhibits interleukin-5 mRNA expression and cysteinyl leukotriene production in ragweed and mite-stimulated peripheral blood mononuclear cells from patients with asthma. *Allergy Asthma Proc* 24 (5), 359-366

Griffith L.G. and Swartz M.A. (2006) Capturing complex 3D tissue physiology *in vitro*

Hasty, P. et al. (1995) Severe phenotype in mice with termination mutation in exon 2 of cystic fibrosis gene. *Somat. Cell Mol. Genet.*, 21, 177–187

Haws C.; Finkbeiner W.E.; Widdicombe J.H.; Wine J.J.; (1994) Calu-3: a human airway epithelial cell line that shows cAMP-dependent Cl- secretion., *Am J Physiol.* 266, 493-501

Henjakovic, M. et al. (2008) Ex vivo lung function measurements in precision-cut lung slices (PCLS) from chemical allergen-sensitized mice represent a suitable alternative to in vivo studies. *Toxicol Sci* 106 (2), 444-453

Hirano K.; Yamashita S.; Kuga Y.; Sakai N.; Nozaki S.; Kihara S.; Arai T.; Yanagi K.; Takami S.; Menju M. (1995) Atherosclerotic disease in marked hyperalphalipoproteinemia. Combined reduction of cholesteryl ester transfer protein and hepatic triglyceride lipase. *Arterioscler Thromb Vasc Biol.* ; 15: 1849–1856

Hofmann, W.; Asgharian, B. and Winkler-Heil, R. (2002). Intersubject variability in particle deposition in human lungs. *J. Aerosol Sci.* 33, 219 –235.

Huang S.; Wiszniewski L.; Derouette J.P.; Constant S. (2009), *In vitro* organ culture models of asthma *Drug Discovery Today: Disease Models* Vol. 6, No. 4

Hubatsch, I.; Ragnarsson, E.G.E. and Artursson, P. (2007) Determination of drug permeability and prediction of drug absorption in Caco-2 monolayers. *Nature Protocols* 2: 2111-2119.

Inazu A.; Brown M.L.; Hesler C.B.; Agellon L.B.; Koizumi J.; Takata K.; Maruhama Y.; Mabuchi H.; Tall A.R. (1990) Increased high-density lipoprotein levels caused by a common cholesteryl-ester transfer protein gene mutation. *N Engl J Med.* 323: 1234–1238

Ishii H. et al. (2005) Alveolar macrophage-epithelial cell interaction following exposure to atmospheric particles induces the release of mediators involved in monocyte mobilization and recruitment. *Respir Res* 6: 87

Ishii N. ; Nakahigashi K.; Baba T.; Robert M. et al. (2007) Multiple High-Throughput Analyses Monitor the Response of E. coli to Perturbations. *Science* 316: 593-597

Karlas A., Machuy N.; ShinY.J.; Pleissner K-P; Artarin A.; Heuer; Becker D.; Khalil H.; Ogilvie LA; Hess S.; Maeurer AP; Müller E.; Wolff T.; Rudel T.; Meyer TF (2010) Genome-wide RNAi screen identifies human host factors crucial for influenza virus replication. *Nature* 463: 818-822

Kerem E.; Corey M.; Gold R.; Levison H. (1990) Pulmonary function and clinical course in patients with cystic fibrosis after pulmonary colonization with Pseudomonas aeruginosa. *J Paediatr;* 116: 714d719

Koizumi, J.; Inazu, A.; Yagi, K.; Koizumi, I.; Uno, Y.; Kajinami, K.; Miyamoto, S.; Moulin, P.; Tall, AR.; Mabuchi, H.; et al. (1991) Serum lipoprotein lipid concentration and composition in homozygous and heterozygous patients with cholesteryl ester transfer protein deficiency. *Atherosclerosis.* 90: 189–196

Laberge, S. and El Bassam, S. (2004) Cytokines, structural cells of the lungs and airway inflammation. *Paediatr. Respir. Rev.* 5 (Suppl. A), S41–45

Lang, D.S. et al. (1998) Interactions between human bronchoepithelial cells and lung fibroblasts after ozone exposure *in vitro. Toxicol Lett* 96-97, 13-24

Mäkelä, M.J.; Puhakka, T.; Ruuskanen, O.; Leinonen, M.; Saikku, P.; Kimpimäki, M.; Blomqvist, S.; Hyypiä, T. and Arstila, P. (1998) Viruses and Bacteria in the Etiology of the Common Cold *J Clin Microbiol.* February; 36(2): 539–542

Matsui H.; Grubb B.R.; Tarran R.; Randell S.H.; Gatzy J.T.; normal Ion Composition, in the Pathogenesis of Cystic Fibrosis Airways Disease. *Cell,* Vol. 95, 1005-1015.

Mögel, M.; Krüger, E.; Krug, H.F.; Seidel, A. (1998) A new coculture-system of bronchial epithelial and endothelial cells as a model for studying ozone effects on airway tissue. *Toxicol. Letter* 96-97, 25-32

Morin, C. et al. (2005) Organ-cultured airway explants: a new model of airway hyperresponsiveness. *Exp Lung Res* 31 (7), 719-744

Nakamura, Y. et al. (2008) Cigarette smoke extract induces thymic stromal lymphopoietin expression, leading to T(H)2-type immune responses and airway inflammation. *J. Allergy Clin. Immunol.* 122, 1208–1214

Neumann, G.; Noda, T. & Kawaoka, Y (2009) Emergence and pandemic potential of swine-origin H1N1 influenza virus. *Nature* 459: 931–939

Nilsson, C. et al. (2004) Low numbers of interleukin-12-producing cord blood mononuclear cells and immunoglobulin E sensitization in early childhood. *Clin Exp Allergy* 34 (3), 373-380

Noble D. (1960) "Cardiac action and pacemaker potentials based on the Hodgkin-Huxley equations". *Nature* 188 (4749): 495–497

Noble D. (2006) The music of life: Biology beyond the genome. *Oxford: Oxford University Press*. pp. 176. ISBN 978-0-19-929573-9

O'Neal, W.K.; Hasty, P.; McCray, P.B.; Casey, B.; Rivera-Perez, J.; Welsh, M.J.; Beaudet, A. and Bradley, A. (1993) A severe phenotype in mice with a duplication of exon 3 in the cystic fibrosis locus. *Hum. Mol. Genet.*, 2, 1561–1569

O'Sullivan, BP.; Freedman, SD (2009) Cystic fibrosis. *Lancet*; 373: 1891–904

Pauwels, RA.; Rabe KF (2004) Burden and clinical features of chronic obstructive pulmonary disease (COPD). *Lancet* 364: 613–620

Plotkin, S.L. and Plotkin, S.A. (2008) "A short history of vaccination." *In: Vaccines*, pp. 6-7

Ratcliff, R.; Evans, M.J.; Cuthbert, A.W.; MacVinish, L.J.; Foster, D.; Anderson, J.R. and Colledge, W.H. (1993) Production of a severe cystic fibrosis mutation in mice by gene targeting. *Nature Genet.*, 4, 35–41

Rich, D.P.; Berger, H.A.; Cheng, S.H.; Travis, S.M.; Saxena, M.; Smith, A.E. and Welsh, M.J. (1993) Regulation of the cystic fibrosis transmembrane conductance regulator Cl – channel by negative charge in the R domain. *J. Biol. Chem.*, 268, 20259–20267

Rochman, Y. and Leonard, W.J. (2008) Thymic stromal lymphopoietin: a new cytokine in asthma. *Curr. Opin. Pharmacol.* 8, 249–254

Santegoets, S.J. et al. (2008) Human dendritic cell line models for DC differentiation and clinical DC vaccination studies. *J Leukoc Biol* 84 (6), 1364-1373

Shi, L. et al. (2008) Local blockade of TSLP receptor alleviated allergic disease by regulating airway dendritic cells. *Clin. Immunol.* 129, 202–210

Singh J et al., Identification of potent and novel alpha4beta1 antagonists using *in silico* screening, *J. Med. Chem.* 45 (2002), pp. 2988–2993

Snouwaert, J.N.; Brigman, K.K.; Latour, A.M.; Malouf, N.N.; Boucher, R.C.; Smithies, O. and Koller, B.H. (1992) An animal model for cystic fibrosis made by gene targeting. *Science*, 257, 1083–1088

Suzuki, S. et al. (2007) Expression of interleukin-17F in a mouse model of allergic asthma. *Int. Arch. Allergy Immunol.* 143 (Suppl 1), 89–94

Tall A. R.; Yvan-Charvet, L.; Wang N. (2007) The Failure of Torcetrapib: Was it the Molecule or the Mechanism? *Arterioscler Thromb Vasc Biol* 27 : 257-260.

Tan, L. et al. (2009) Immunomodulatory effect of cytosine-phosphate-guanosine (CpG)-oligonucleotides in nonasthmatic chronic rhinosinusitis: an explant model. *Am J Rhinol Allergy* 23 (2), 123-129

Tang, L. et al. (2003) Expression and characterization of recombinant canine IL-13 receptor alpha2 protein and its biological activity *in vitro*. *Mol Immunol* 39 (12), 719-727

Ugwoke, M.I.; Agu, R.U.; Verbeke, N. and Kinget, R. (2005) Nasal mucoadhesive drug delivery: Background, applications, trends and future perspectives. *Advanced Drug Delivery Reviews* 57, 1640-1665

Van Riel D.; Munster V.J.; De Wit E.; et al. H5N1 attachment to lower respiratory tract. *Science* 2006; 312 : 399

Verstraelen, S. et al. (2008) Cell types involved in allergic asthma and their use in *in vitro* models to assess respiratory sensitization. *Toxicol. In vitro* 22, 1419–1431

Von Bertalanffy L. (1968) General System theory: Foundations, Development, Applications. George Braziller. pp. 295. ISBN 9780807604533.

Welsh M.J. and Smith A. E. (1995) "Cystic Fibrosis." *Scientific American* 273 (6): 52-59.

Wohlsen, A. et al. (2003) The early allergic response in small airways of human precision-cut lung slices. *Eur Respir J* 21 (6), 1024-1032

Wong, C.K. et al. (2005) Role of p38 MAPK and NF-kB for chemokine release in coculture of human eosinophils and bronchial epithelial cells. *Clin Exp Immunol* 139 (1), 90-100

Ying, S. et al. (2005) Thymic stromal lymphopoietin expression is increased in asthmatic airways and correlates with expression of Th2-attracting chemokines and disease severity. *J. Immunol.* 174, 8183–8190

Yoo, J. et al. (2005) Spontaneous atopic dermatitis in mice expressing an inducible thymic stromal lymphopoietin transgene specifically in the skin. *J. Exp. Med.* 202, 541–549

Zaph, C. et al. (2007) Epithelial-cell-intrinsic IKK-beta expression regulates intestinal immune homeostasis. *Nature* 446, 552–556

Ziegler, S.F. and Liu, Y.J. (2006) Thymic stromal lymphopoietin in normal and pathogenic T cell development and function. *Nat. Immunol.* 7, 709–714

Zhou, B. et al. (2005) Thymic stromal lymphopoietin as a key initiator of allergic airway inflammation in mice. *Nat. Immunol.* 6, 1047–1053

Permissions

The contributors of this book come from diverse backgrounds, making this book a truly international effort. This book will bring forth new frontiers with its revolutionizing research information and detailed analysis of the nascent developments around the world.

We would like to thank Izet M. Kapetanovic, for lending his expertise to make the book truly unique. He has played a crucial role in the development of this book. Without his invaluable contribution this book wouldn't have been possible. He has made vital efforts to compile up to date information on the varied aspects of this subject to make this book a valuable addition to the collection of many professionals and students.

This book was conceptualized with the vision of imparting up-to-date information and advanced data in this field. To ensure the same, a matchless editorial board was set up. Every individual on the board went through rigorous rounds of assessment to prove their worth. After which they invested a large part of their time researching and compiling the most relevant data for our readers. Conferences and sessions were held from time to time between the editorial board and the contributing authors to present the data in the most comprehensible form. The editorial team has worked tirelessly to provide valuable and valid information to help people across the globe.

Every chapter published in this book has been scrutinized by our experts. Their significance has been extensively debated. The topics covered herein carry significant findings which will fuel the growth of the discipline. They may even be implemented as practical applications or may be referred to as a beginning point for another development. Chapters in this book were first published by InTech; hereby published with permission under the Creative Commons Attribution License or equivalent.

The editorial board has been involved in producing this book since its inception. They have spent rigorous hours researching and exploring the diverse topics which have resulted in the successful publishing of this book. They have passed on their knowledge of decades through this book. To expedite this challenging task, the publisher supported the team at every step. A small team of assistant editors was also appointed to further simplify the editing procedure and attain best results for the readers.

Our editorial team has been hand-picked from every corner of the world. Their multi-ethnicity adds dynamic inputs to the discussions which result in innovative outcomes. These outcomes are then further discussed with the researchers and contributors who give their valuable feedback and opinion regarding the same. The feedback is then collaborated with the researches and they are edited in a comprehensive manner to aid the understanding of the subject.

Apart from the editorial board, the designing team has also invested a significant amount of their time in understanding the subject and creating the most relevant covers. They scrutinized every image to scout for the most suitable representation of the subject and create an appropriate cover for the book.

The publishing team has been involved in this book since its early stages. They were actively engaged in every process, be it collecting the data, connecting with the contributors or procuring relevant information. The team has been an ardent support to the editorial, designing and production team. Their endless efforts to recruit the best for this project, has resulted in the accomplishment of this book. They are a veteran in the field of academics and their pool of knowledge is as vast as their experience in printing. Their expertise and guidance has proved useful at every step. Their uncompromising quality standards have made this book an exceptional effort. Their encouragement from time to time has been an inspiration for everyone.

The publisher and the editorial board hope that this book will prove to be a valuable piece of knowledge for researchers, students, practitioners and scholars across the globe.

List of Contributors

Izet M. Kapetanovic
Division of Cancer Prevention, National Cancer Institute, Bethesda, MD, USA

Pierre M. Durand and Theresa L. Coetzer
University of the Witwatersrand and National Health Laboratory Service, South Africa

Klaus Pors
Institute of Cancer Therapeutics, University of Bradford, UK

Bhushan Patwardhan
Symbiosis International University, Pune

Kapil Khambholja
Novartis Healthcare Pvt. Limited, Hyderabad, India

C.R. Lemech and H.T. Arkenau
Sarah Cannon Research UK, London, UK
Cancer Institute, University College London, UK

R.S. Kristeleit
Cancer Institute, University College London, UK

Celia Gellman, Susana Mingote, Yvonne Wang and Stephen Rayport
Department of Psychiatry, Columbia University
Department of Molecular Therapeutics, New York State Psychiatric Institute

Inna Gaisler-Salomon
Department of Psychology, University of Haifa, USA
Department of Psychiatry, Columbia University

Sergio Y. Alcoser and Melinda G. Hollingshead
Biological Testing Branch, Developmental Therapeutics Program, National Cancer Institute, USA

Albert P. Li
In Vitro ADMET Laboratories LLC and Advanced Pharmaceutical Sciences Inc., Columbia, MD, USA

Song Huang, Ludovic Wiszniewski and Samuel Constant
Epithelix Sàrl, Switzerland